Barbara O'Neill's inspired essential
Tricks for Daily Wellness: Simple Recipes,
Natural Health and Wellbeing Tips.

Volume 1

Disclaimer and/or Legal Notices

The content presented in this book is for educational and informational purposes only. While I am not a medical professional, the information compiled in this book reflects thorough research and diligent effort to present accurate interpretations of Barbara O'Neill's teachings and education. However, this book is not intended as medical advice, nor should it replace consultation with a healthcare professional.

The insights and strategies shared in this book are based on my understanding and experiences, alongside comprehensive research into Barbara O'Neill's methodologies. The recommendations and advice are intended for healthy adults. Before adopting any of the practices, remedies, or suggestions contained within this book, it is crucial to consult with your physician, particularly if you have any existing health conditions or concerns.

I have endeavored to ensure the accuracy and reliability of the information provided, but it should be noted that the field of natural health is continuously evolving. Thus, some information may become outdated or be interpreted differently as new research emerges. If any errors or inaccuracies are found within this text, I warmly welcome feedback and corrections. Please feel free to contact me via email for any suggestions or to address potential updates in future editions of this book.

This book is intended to share knowledge and inspire a holistic approach to health and wellness. However, the author does not assume responsibility for any consequences, real or perceived, from applying the information herein. Your support and constructive feedback on our page are highly appreciated, whether it be positive reinforcement or critical insights. Your input is invaluable in our mission to provide valuable and accurate content to all readers interested in natural healing and Barbara O'Neill's teachings.

A Better You Everyday Publications
email address abetteryoueveryday2022@gmail.com

www.abetteryoueveryday.com

Barbara O'Neill's inspired essential Tricks for Daily Wellness: Simple Recipes, Natural Health and Wellbeing Tips

From Kitchen to Lifestyle: Transforming Everyday Routines into Balanced, Joyful Living

By Margaret Willowbrook

Volume 1

USA

2024

TABLE OF CONTENTS

FOREWORD.

In the tranquil embrace of nature, amidst the rustling leaves and the whispering winds, lies a reservoir of timeless wisdom waiting to be discovered. It is with immense joy and a profound sense of responsibility that I present to you this compendium of insights, a reflection of the endless possibilities that nature offers for healing, balance, and well-being. This book is not merely a collection of writings; it is a mosaic of knowledge, carefully pieced together to guide you towards a life steeped in harmony and health.

The inspiration for this eclectic collection springs from the teachings and philosophy of Barbara O'Neill, a figure synonymous with harnessing nature's wisdom for health and vitality. Her approach, blending the simplicity of natural living with the profundity of holistic health, sets the tone for the diverse topics you will encounter in this book. Like Barbara, we believe in the transformative power of nature's remedies and lifestyle choices that prioritize balance and wellness.

In these pages, you will find echoes of Barbara's philosophy, translated into practical and accessible knowledge. Her influence is a golden thread that weaves through each topic, be it a simple recipe, a wellness tip, or a deep dive into natural health. Her teachings remind us that the most profound healing often comes from the simplest sources; the foods we eat, the air we breathe, and the routines we follow.

This book is a tribute to Barbara O'Neill's vision; a vision where health is approached holistically, and daily practices are imbued with the wisdom of nature. Each section, while unique in its focus, embodies this holistic approach, inviting you to explore the many facets of wellness and how they harmoniously interconnect in our lives.

As you embark on the journey through these pages, you are not just reading a book; you are embarking on a pilgrimage. A pilgrimage that will take you through the verdant valleys of herbal wisdom, across the serene landscapes of traditional practices, and into the bustling streets of the modern world, laden with pragmatic, everyday applications. This book is more than a guide; it is a companion on your odyssey towards a life of vitality and equilibrium.

In an era where the relentless pace of modernity often drowns out the gentle whispers of natural intuition, this book aspires to be a bridge. A bridge that spans the gap between the enduring wisdom of yesteryears and the pressing demands of contemporary life. It is a pathway that leads you back to the essence of true wellness, where ancient knowledge and present-day realities converge in a harmonious symphony.

The genesis of this collection lies in a deep reverence for the Earth's bounty and an unwavering belief in the curative prowess of the natural world. It is a tribute to the idea that within the simplicity of nature lies the secret to health, contentment, and a tranquility that transcends the physical realm. Each chapter, each topic, is steeped in this ethos, beckoning you to explore, absorb, and transform.

As you go through these pages, I invite you to open not just your mind but also your heart to the myriad possibilities that lie within. May you find in these words the spark to embrace a more natural way of living, the bravery to initiate changes that resonate with your soul, and the insight to maintain equilibrium in all facets of life.

Welcome to a voyage of discovery, healing, and communion with the subtle yet profound power of nature.

This book is akin to a gentle stream, meandering through the landscapes of natural healing and holistic wellness. It is a stream fed by countless tributaries; each article, each piece of advice, contributing to the flow of knowledge and understanding. As you navigate these waters, you will encounter the confluence of tradition and innovation, of ancient practices and modern research. Here, the wisdom of the past is not forgotten but is instead reimagined and reintegrated into the tapestry of contemporary life.

In these chapters, you will find a celebration of the diversity and richness of nature's offerings. From the humble kitchen ingredients that hold secret healing powers to the elaborate rituals that promise to soothe the soul and invigorate the body, each topic is a testament to the multifaceted nature of health and wellness. You will be introduced to practices that have stood the test of time, remedies passed down through generations, and innovations that bring a fresh perspective to age-old challenges.

But this book is more than a repository of knowledge. It is an invitation to engage in a dialogue with yourself and with the world around you. It is an encouragement to observe, to experiment, and to experience. Each topic is presented not as a prescriptive solution but as a starting point for exploration and self-discovery. The practices and insights offered here are not meant to be followed blindly but are to be adapted to your unique journey towards wellness.

This journey is as much about the destination as it is about the path. It is about finding joy in the small rituals, appreciating the subtle changes, and celebrating the milestones. It is about learning to listen to your body, to understand its language, and to respond with love and care. This book encourages you to slow down, to breathe deeply, and to reconnect with the innate wisdom that lies within and all around you.

As you traverse through these topics, you may find that what begins as a quest for physical health gradually transforms into a deeper quest for a more fulfilling, more connected way of life. You will discover that wellness is not a static state but a dynamic process, one that involves continuous learning, adapting, and growing. You will learn that health is not just about the absence of disease but about the presence of vitality, joy, and a deep sense of well-being.

This collection of writings aims to empower you. It seeks to provide you with the tools and knowledge to take charge of your health, to make informed choices, and to cultivate practices that nourish and sustain you. It is a guide that respects your individuality, acknowledges your unique challenges and aspirations, and offers support and guidance on your path to wellness.

As you embark on this journey, remember that you are not alone. You are part of a community of seekers, of individuals who are striving to live more consciously, more healthfully, and more in tune with nature. This book is a reflection of that collective quest; a quest for balance, for harmony, and for a life lived in alignment with the natural rhythms of the world.

In conclusion, this book is an ode to the enduring wisdom of nature and the resilience of the human spirit. It is a celebration of the small, everyday choices that lead to big transformations. It is a reminder that in every leaf, in every drop of water, in every breath of air, lies the potential for healing and renewal. May this book be a source of inspiration, a beacon of hope, and a companion on your journey towards a life of true wellness.

Welcome to a world where every step is a step towards balance, every word a seed of wisdom, and every practice a pathway to a life of harmony and health. Welcome to the journey of a lifetime.

INTRODUCTION.

Welcome to a journey that defies the conventional, a journey where each step is an adventure, and every page turn opens a window to a new horizon of knowledge and understanding. This book is not just a compilation of health and wellness topics; it's a kaleidoscope of wisdom, each piece distinct yet contributing to a grand, colorful pattern of holistic well-being.

Barbara O'Neill's influence is palpable in the structure and spirit of this book. Her philosophy advocates for simplicity and accessibility in achieving wellness, a principle that is the cornerstone of each topic you'll encounter here. Barbara's teachings inspire us to look at health not as a distant goal but as an accessible, daily journey; one that is enriched by every small, mindful choice we make.

As you navigate through the variety of topics, you will experience the essence of Barbara's guidance; the understanding that every individual's path to wellness is unique, and that the wisdom of nature has something for everyone. This book is designed to reflect that philosophy, offering a diverse range of topics to cater to the myriad paths of personal health journeys.

The structure of this book, resembling a collection of short, insightful topics, mirrors Barbara's approach to teaching; where each piece of knowledge is presented as an integral part of a larger, cohesive picture of health and well-being. Just as Barbara's teachings span a wide range of subjects, so too does this book, offering a holistic view of wellness.

In this way, the book stands as a tribute to Barbara O'Neill's enduring wisdom. It invites you to embark on your wellness journey with the same spirit of curiosity and openness that she championed. Each topic, a steppingstone on this path, encourages you to embrace the simplicity and effectiveness of natural health and wellness, just as Barbara has taught us.

The structure of this book is intentionally designed to be like a vibrant mosaic. Each topic stands alone, a complete picture in itself, yet contributing to the broader image of health and wellness. This approach mirrors the very nature of life; diverse, surprising, and richly varied. It's akin to a stroll through a lush garden, where each step brings you to a different plant, each with its own unique beauty and benefits.

Why have we chosen this structure? Because we understand that the journey to health and well-being is not linear. It's a path filled with turns and twists, with new discoveries waiting around each bend. This book allows you to meander through the garden of wellness, stopping to admire a flower here, to pick a fruit there, each time adding something valuable to your basket of knowledge.

Each topic in this book is a world in itself, an island of information where you can dock your boat and explore. Like an explorer charting unknown territories, you can navigate these topics in any order, at any pace, according to your interests and needs. This book is your atlas, with each topic a destination offering its unique landscape and treasures.

The beauty of this approach is its flexibility. Whether you have a specific health concern in mind or are just browsing for interesting reads, this book caters to both needs. It's like a box of assorted chocolates; each piece offers a different flavor, and you can choose what appeals to you at the moment.

This book is meant to be fun, engaging, and educational. Just as a child flips through a picture book, delighted by the images that catch their eye, you too can flip through these pages, finding joy and interest in the topics that resonate with you. Each article is crafted to be both informative and enjoyable, combining the light-heartedness of a leisurely read with the depth of a scholarly article.

We understand that in today's fast-paced world, taking time to read a book cover to cover is a luxury many cannot afford. This book respects your time and attention. It's designed for the reader who wants to learn something new about health and wellness without committing to a lengthy read. It's for the morning commuter, the busy parent, the student on a break; anyone who seeks a quick yet enriching read.

You can see this book as a friendly companion on a lazy Sunday afternoon, or as a reliable resource on a busy weekday. It's your go-to for health tips while sipping your morning coffee or for a relaxing read before bed. This book fits into your life, adapting to your schedule and interests, always ready to offer something new and exciting.

Moreover, this format invites spontaneity and surprise. Just as life is unpredictable, so are the pages of this book. You might open it seeking information on herbal teas and find yourself captivated by an article on the health benefits of laughter. This serendipitous exploration is one of the joys of this book, mirroring the unpredictable yet delightful journey of life itself.

This book also serves as a reminder that health and wellness are not just about rigid diets and strict exercise regimes. It's about finding joy in the little things, learning new facts about the world around us, and understanding how our bodies and minds work in harmony with nature. Each topic offers a chance to pause, reflect, and perhaps even smile at the wonders of our natural world.

In creating this book, we envisioned a resource that would stand the test of time, a book that you could return to again and again, always finding something new and relevant. It's a living document, evolving with your journey through life, adapting to your changing interests and needs.

In summary, this book is an invitation to a dance, a dance through the myriad aspects of health and wellness, where each step is a discovery, and each turn is a new opportunity to learn and grow. It's an open invitation to celebrate the diversity of natural health, to embrace the joy of learning, and to weave your own unique pattern in the rich fabric of holistic well-being.

So, open this book at any page, start your journey anywhere, and let the adventure begin. Welcome to a world of health, happiness, and discovery; a world where every read is a delight and every topic a treasure.

ONION SOCKS: AN UNEXPECTED COLD REMEDY.

In the enchanting world of home remedies, where nature's pantry offers solutions to our everyday ailments, there lies a remedy as curious as it is charming; the practice of placing onion slices in one's socks at bedtime. It's a tradition that might raise eyebrows or evoke a chuckle, but delve a little deeper, and you'll discover a tapestry of wisdom, tradition, and perhaps a touch of unexpected science. Let us look deeply into this quaint yet fascinating remedy and unravel the mysteries of onion socks.

THE ROOTS OF THE REMEDY: A NOD TO TRADITION AND BARBARA O'NEILL'S TEACHINGS.

The idea of tucking onion slices into one's socks might seem like a page taken from an old wives' tale, but it's grounded in a holistic understanding of health. This practice aligns beautifully with the teachings of natural health advocates like Barbara O'Neill, who have always emphasized the importance of using nature's offerings for healing. The onion, humble in its presence, is a powerhouse of medicinal properties, and this remedy is a testament to the age-old belief in nature's ability to heal.

UNDERSTANDING THE ONION'S POWER.

Onions are more than just a staple in the kitchen; they are a storehouse of antibacterial, anti-inflammatory, and antiviral properties. Rich in sulfur-containing compounds and quercetin, onions have been used for centuries to combat infections and boost immunity. It's this very potency that makes the onion an interesting choice for a remedy that's as simple as it is intriguing.

9

The Concept of Reflexology and Detoxification.

The practice of placing onions in socks draws on the principles of reflexology, a discipline that views the feet as mirrors to the body's internal health. Each area of the foot is believed to correspond to different organs and bodily systems. Placing onions against the soles, therefore, is thought to facilitate a kind of detoxification, where the onion absorbs toxins and purifies the blood. While modern science may offer a skeptical eyebrow to this claim, the anecdotal evidence and the persistence of this remedy through generations lend it a certain charm and intrigue.

A Natural Approach to Cold and Flu Prevention.

The onion-sock remedy is often hailed as a preventive measure against colds and flu. The logic is twofold: firstly, the natural compounds in onions, like quercetin and sulfur, are believed to strengthen the immune system. Secondly, the warmth generated by wearing socks during sleep is thought to promote circulation, further aiding in the body's ability to ward off infections.

The Placebo Effect: More Than Meets the Eye.

Skeptics might attribute the effectiveness of onion socks to the placebo effect; the power of belief. But in healing, the placebo effect has its place. If a ritual, as simple as placing onions in one's socks, brings comfort, induces relaxation, and promotes a sense of well-being, then it serves a purpose. After all, the mind's influence over the body's health is a terrain that modern science continues to explore with fascination.

Trying the Onion Sock Remedy.

For the curious and the health-conscious, trying this remedy is a simple and safe adventure into the world of traditional wellness practices. Before bedtime, take a fresh, clean onion and slice it thinly. Place a slice or two inside each sock and wear them as you sleep. The idea is to let the onions sit against the soles of your feet, working their supposed magic throughout the night.

A Journey into Wholesome Sleep.

Beyond its purported physical benefits, the onion sock remedy invites a ritualistic approach to bedtime. In a world where the end of the day often means collapsing into bed with a mind full of the day's worries, this remedy offers a moment of pause, a ritual that marks the transition from wakefulness to sleep. It's a practice that encourages mindfulness and care, a nightly act of self-nurturing that aligns well with Barbara O'Neill's teachings of holistic well-being.

Embracing the Quirky with Open Arms.

While the practice of sleeping with onion slices in your socks may not boast a robust backing from scientific research, it stands as a harmless, intriguing remedy with roots in traditional wellness practices. Whether it's the potential health benefits of the onion, the placebo effect, or simply the comforting ritual that appeals, it's a unique tradition that's worth exploring for those inclined towards natural health practices.

In the grand scheme of wellness, remedies like onion socks remind us of the beauty and simplicity inherent in many traditional practices. Who knows, this quirky bedtime tradition might just surprise you with its soothing touch, adding an unexpected yet delightful twist to your nightly routine.

THE QUICK AT-HOME TEETH WHITENING SECRET.

In the quest for a brighter smile, many turn to expensive treatments and chemical-laden products, often overlooking the treasures hidden in the simplicity of our everyday lives. Among these hidden gems is a surprisingly effective and quick at-home teeth whitening secret. This secret, rooted in both traditional wisdom and a dash of modern understanding, offers a light-hearted and educational journey into natural dental care.

THE QUEST FOR WHITER TEETH: A MODERN OBSESSION.

In today's image-conscious society, a bright smile is often seen as a symbol of health and vitality. It's no wonder that teeth whitening has become a burgeoning industry. Amidst this rush towards commercial solutions, the teachings of natural health advocates like Barbara O'Neill remind us of the power and simplicity of nature's remedies. She has always championed natural approaches to health, emphasizing the need to turn to nature for answers. This approach is not just about effectiveness but also about understanding and respecting our bodies by choosing safer, more natural methods.

UNLOCKING THE SECRET: NATURE'S INGREDIENTS.

The secret to at-home teeth whitening lies in some common, yet powerful, natural ingredients. These components, often found in our kitchens, have been used for centuries to maintain oral health and hygiene. Unlike commercial whiteners, these natural alternatives are gentle, devoid of harsh chemicals, and kind to your enamel.

Baking Soda: The Gentle Abrasive.

Baking soda, a common household item, plays a starring role in natural teeth whitening. Its mild abrasive properties help gently scrub away surface stains on the teeth, making it a popular ingredient in many natural toothpaste recipes. When used correctly, baking soda can help restore the natural whiteness of your teeth without the harshness of chemical whiteners.

Hydrogen Peroxide: Nature's Disinfectant.

Hydrogen peroxide, another common household item, is known for its natural bleaching and disinfecting properties. When used in small quantities, it can aid in lightening teeth stains. It's the same ingredient used in many commercial whitening products, but at home, you can control its concentration and usage, making it a safer alternative for occasional use.

The Lemon Juice Debate.

Lemon juice is often touted as a natural whitening agent due to its acidic properties. However, caution is advised. While it can help in removing stains, its high acidity can also erode tooth enamel over time. This is a reminder of the importance of balance and moderation in natural remedies; a principle often highlighted in Barbara O'Neill's teachings.

Coconut Oil: An Ancient Practice Revisited.

Oil pulling, an ancient practice involving swishing oil in the mouth, has seen a resurgence in popularity. Coconut oil, with its pleasant taste and antimicrobial properties, is a favorite choice. This technique is believed to pull toxins from the mouth, improve oral health, and consequently, brighten the teeth.

A Practical Guide to At-Home Whitening.

To harness these natural ingredients for teeth whitening, one can adopt simple practices at home. A mixture of baking soda and water, applied gently with a toothbrush, can serve as an effective weekly treatment. For those opting to use hydrogen peroxide, a diluted rinse can be used sparingly to avoid overuse. Coconut oil pulling can be incorporated into daily routines, swishing the oil in the mouth for about 15 minutes before brushing.

Words of Caution.

While these natural methods are gentle and effective, it's crucial to approach them with care. Overuse of any abrasive, including baking soda, or misuse of acidic substances, can harm your enamel. As with all health practices, moderation is key.

Beyond Whitening: Embracing Holistic Oral Health.

Barbara O'Neill's philosophy extends beyond mere appearance, emphasizing overall health and well-being. This approach to teeth whitening is not just about aesthetics but is part of a holistic view of health. Maintaining good oral hygiene, eating a balanced diet, and regular dental check-ups are integral to this holistic approach.

A Smile That Reflects Natural Health.

In embracing this quick at-home teeth whitening secret, you are doing more than just brightening your smile; you are taking a step towards natural, holistic health practices. This journey into the world of natural oral care is not just a means to an end but a delightful exploration of what nature has to offer. It reminds us that sometimes, the most effective solutions are the simplest ones, waiting to be rediscovered in our own homes.

Tasty Salads That Naturally Aid Weight Loss.

In the colorful world of healthy eating, salads have long been cherished as allies in weight loss and wellness journeys. But, let's dispel the myth: salads need not be bland or monotonous. In fact, the secret to a satisfying, weight-loss-friendly salad lies in its ability to be both delicious and nutritionally balanced. This exploration into tasty salads is not just about shedding pounds; it's about embracing a joyful way of eating that aligns with Barbara O'Neill's teachings of natural health and wellbeing.

The Art of Crafting a Weight-Loss Salad.

Creating a salad that aids in weight loss while tantalizing your taste buds is an art. It's about mixing textures, colors, and flavors to create a dish that's as appealing to the eyes as it is to the palate. The key lies in selecting ingredients that are low in calories but high in nutrients; a principle often echoed in Barbara O'Neill's approach to holistic health.

Greens: The Foundation.

Start with a variety of fresh greens; spinach, kale, arugula, and romaine are excellent choices. Greens are not only low in calories but also packed with fiber, vitamins, and minerals. Fiber is particularly important as it helps you feel full longer, reducing the tendency to snack on less healthy options.

Protein: The Powerhouse.

Incorporating lean protein is essential for a salad that supports weight loss. It helps build muscle and keeps you feeling satiated. Consider adding grilled chicken, tofu, legumes, or boiled eggs. For those who follow Barbara O'Neill's teachings, which often emphasize plant-based sources, chickpeas, black beans, and lentils are not only protein-rich but also add a wonderful texture to your salad.

COLORFUL VEGETABLES AND FRUITS: THE FLAVOR BOOSTERS.

Vegetables and fruits add a burst of color, flavor, and vital nutrients without many calories. Carrots, bell peppers, cucumbers, tomatoes, and berries are excellent choices. They bring in antioxidants and vitamins, crucial for overall health and wellness. Remember, the more colorful your salad, the wider the range of nutrients.

HEALTHY FATS: THE SATISFYING TOUCH.

Don't shy away from fats! Healthy fats are essential for nutrient absorption and can make your salad more satisfying. Avocado, nuts, seeds, and olive oil are great options. They add creaminess and crunch, making your salad a well-rounded meal.

DRESSINGS: THE HEART OF FLAVOR.

Salads often get a bad reputation from calorie-laden dressings. Opt for homemade dressings using olive oil, lemon juice, herbs, and spices. A simple vinaigrette or a yogurt-based dressing can provide flavor without the excess calories of store-bought dressings.

PORTION CONTROL: THE HIDDEN SECRET.

Even the healthiest salad can contribute to weight gain if eaten in large quantities. Barbara O'Neill advocates for mindful eating, which includes being aware of portions. Listen to your body's hunger cues and avoid eating out of habit or boredom.

THE ROLE OF HERBS AND SPICES.

Herbs and spices are unsung heroes in making salads exciting. Basil, mint, cilantro, and dill can transform your dish. Spices like cumin, paprika, and black pepper not only add flavor but also have metabolism-boosting properties.

HYDRATION: AN ESSENTIAL COMPANION.

Accompany your salad with plenty of water. Staying hydrated is crucial for weight loss and overall health. Herbal teas or infused water with lemon, cucumber, or mint can be refreshing options that support your weight loss efforts.

EXPERIMENTATION: THE KEY TO ENJOYMENT.

The beauty of salads lies in their versatility. Experiment with different ingredients, textures, and dressings. Keeping your salads varied will not only keep your taste buds happy but also ensure a wider range of nutrients.

A CELEBRATION OF FLAVORS AND HEALTH.

Salads for weight loss need not be a mundane affair. They can be a delightful exploration of flavors and textures, a testament to the joy of eating healthily. Embracing salads as part of your weight loss journey is about celebrating fresh, natural ingredients, the very elements that Barbara O'Neill often highlights in her teachings. It's about finding pleasure in the simplicity and richness of nature's bounty.

Natural Hair Care: Herbal Secrets for Healthy Locks.

In the pursuit of healthy, vibrant hair, nature's garden offers a plethora of herbs and natural ingredients, each with its unique properties to nurture and revitalize our locks. This journey into natural hair care is not just about avoiding chemicals; it's a delightful exploration of traditional herbal wisdom, blended with modern understanding, to provide practical, effective solutions for a range of hair concerns.

The Herbal Legacy in Hair Care.

For centuries, people have turned to nature for solutions to their hair woes. Long before the advent of modern hair care products, herbs, and natural ingredients were the go-to solutions for maintaining healthy hair. Barbara O'Neill, an advocate for natural health and healing, often emphasizes the importance of turning to nature for our body's needs, and hair care is no exception. Her teachings encourage exploring herbal remedies, highlighting how they can offer gentle yet effective care for our hair.

Understanding Your Hair's Needs.

The first step in embracing natural hair care is understanding your hair type and its specific needs. Dry, oily, damaged, or normal; each hair type benefits from different herbs and natural treatments. For instance, dry hair may require more moisturizing ingredients like aloe vera or coconut oil, while oily hair may benefit from clarifying herbs like rosemary or mint.

Herbs: Nature's Hair Care Marvels.

Numerous herbs are renowned for their benefits to hair health. Let's explore some of the most celebrated ones:

- Aloe Vera: Known for its soothing and moisturizing properties, aloe vera is excellent for nourishing dry hair and soothing scalp irritations.

- Rosemary: Stimulating hair growth and adding shine, rosemary is a wonder herb for hair revitalization.

- Lavender: With its delightful fragrance, lavender not only promotes hair growth but also reduces stress, a common cause of hair problems.

- Nettle: Rich in minerals and vitamins, nettle helps in combating hair loss and promoting scalp health.

- Hibiscus: Often used in hair masks, hibiscus is known for its ability to enhance hair growth and prevent premature graying.

CREATING YOUR HERBAL HAIR CARE REGIMEN.

Building a natural hair care routine is about integrating these herbs into your daily hair care practices. You can create herbal infusions, hair masks, or even incorporate these herbs into your homemade shampoos and conditioners.

HERBAL INFUSIONS FOR RINSING.

Herbal rinses are an easy way to infuse your hair care routine with the goodness of herbs. Boil water with your herb of choice, strain, and let it cool. Use this infusion as a final rinse after shampooing to reap its benefits. For instance, a chamomile rinse can bring out natural highlights, while a rosemary rinse can boost hair growth.

NOURISHING HAIR MASKS.

Mix herbs with natural ingredients like yogurt, honey, or eggs to create nourishing hair masks. A mask with hibiscus and coconut oil can be a wonderful treat for dry, brittle hair. Apply the mask, leave it on for some time, and then wash off with a gentle, natural shampoo.

Homemade Herbal Shampoos and Conditioners.

For those who love DIY, creating your own herbal shampoos and conditioners can be a fulfilling experience. Blend herbs with natural soap bases or use ingredients like apple cider vinegar for a natural conditioner. The key is to experiment and find what works best for your hair type.

The Importance of a Balanced Diet.

Barbara O'Neill often emphasizes the role of diet in overall health, and hair is no exception. A diet rich in fruits, vegetables, proteins, and healthy fats provides the nutrients necessary for healthy hair growth. Incorporating foods rich in vitamins A, C, E, and minerals like zinc and iron can significantly improve hair health.

Gentle Care and Patience.

Transitioning to natural hair care requires patience. Natural remedies may take longer to show results, but their benefits are long-lasting and without the side effects of harsh chemicals. Handle your hair gently, avoid excessive heat styling, and give your hair the time to adjust to the new, natural regimen.

Embracing Nature's Bounty.

Natural hair care is about more than just maintaining healthy hair; it's about embracing a lifestyle that is in harmony with nature. It encourages us to respect the natural world and its ability to nourish and heal.

THE TRAMPOLINE WORKOUT: FUN FITNESS REVOLUTION.

Bouncing your way to fitness might sound like child's play, but the trampoline workout is a thrilling revolution in the world of exercise, combining the joys of childhood with the rigor of a workout. It's a delightful blend of fun and fitness, bringing a touch of playfulness to the sometimes-monotonous routine of staying in shape.

JUMPING INTO A HEALTHIER LIFESTYLE.

The essence of trampoline workouts lies in their simplicity and effectiveness. Just like Barbara O'Neil often emphasized the importance of finding joy in our health routines, trampoline workouts epitomize this philosophy. This form of exercise turns a fitness session into a playful experience, making it something to look forward to rather than a chore.

THE SCIENCE BEHIND THE BOUNCE.

Bouncing on a trampoline, also known as rebounding, is not just fun but is packed with health benefits. It's a low-impact exercise that is gentle on the joints, making it suitable for all ages and fitness levels. The act of jumping engages multiple muscle groups, enhances coordination, and improves cardiovascular health. It's a holistic workout that nourishes the body, mind, and spirit.

THE BENEFITS: BEYOND JUST FITNESS.

Trampoline workouts offer a myriad of health benefits:

- Lymphatic Flow and Detoxification: Rebounding stimulates the lymphatic system, aiding in the body's detoxification process. It's a natural way to flush out toxins, boosting overall health.

- Bone Health and Strength: The gentle impact of jumping strengthens the bones and increases bone density, making it an excellent exercise for preventing osteoporosis.

- Cardiovascular Improvement: Just like a brisk walk or a run, rebounding gets the heart pumping, improving cardiovascular health without the stress on the legs and feet that comes from hitting the pavement.

- Balance and Coordination: Navigating the unstable surface of a trampoline enhances balance and coordination, skills that are beneficial in every stage of life.

- Stress Relief: The sheer joy of bouncing can reduce stress and elevate mood. The release of endorphins during a trampoline workout can bring about a sense of well-being and happiness.

INCORPORATING TRAMPOLINE WORKOUTS INTO YOUR ROUTINE.

Getting started with trampoline workouts is easy:

- Choose the Right Equipment: Invest in a good quality mini-trampoline with a sturdy frame and responsive springs or bungee cords.

- Start Slow: Begin with basic bouncing and gradually incorporate jumps, twists, and other movements as you get more comfortable.

- Safety First: Ensure you have enough space around the trampoline, and consider using a handlebar for extra stability, especially if you're new to rebounding.

- Mix It Up: Combine trampoline exercises with strength training or yoga for a well-rounded fitness routine.

- Have Fun: The most crucial aspect of a trampoline workout is to have fun. Put on your favorite music and enjoy the bounce.

A JOYFUL PATH TO WELLNESS.

Trampoline workouts represent a joyful path to wellness, aligning perfectly with the philosophy of finding pleasure in maintaining health. It's a testament to the fact that staying fit doesn't have to be tedious or punishing. By doing this, you embark on a delightful journey to health, one that nurtures not just the body but also the soul. The trampoline workout is indeed a revolution, one that brings back the simplicity and joy of youthful play, proving that sometimes, the best way to move forward is to jump up and enjoy the ride.

BEETROOT'S HIDDEN BENEFITS FOR BLOOD PRESSURE AND ENERGY.

The humble beetroot stands out not just for its vivid color but for its remarkable health benefits, particularly for blood pressure management and energy enhancement. This exploration into beetroot's potential is an enjoyable journey through traditional knowledge and modern scientific discovery, showcasing how this root vegetable can be a key player in our wellness regimen.

BEETROOT: A COLORFUL HISTORY AND NUTRITIONAL POWERHOUSE.

Beetroot, with its deep crimson hue, has been a part of human diets for millennia. Historically valued for its medicinal properties, it's now gaining recognition in the scientific community for its health benefits. Barbara O'Neill, often emphasizes the importance of including nutrient-rich foods like beetroot in our diet. This is not only for their ability to address specific health concerns but also for their overall contribution to a balanced and healthy lifestyle.

THE BLOOD PRESSURE CONNECTION.

One of beetroot's most significant health benefits is its ability to help regulate blood pressure. This is primarily due to its high nitrate content. Nitrates are compounds that, once ingested, convert into nitric oxide, a molecule that plays a crucial role in relaxing and dilating blood vessels, thereby improving blood flow and lowering blood pressure.

Numerous studies have shown that consuming beetroot juice can lead to modest reductions in blood pressure. This is particularly beneficial for individuals struggling with hypertension, offering a natural, dietary approach to managing their condition.

BEETROOT FOR ENHANCED ENERGY AND STAMINA.

In addition to its blood pressure-lowering effects, beetroot is also hailed for its ability to boost energy and endurance. This is especially relevant for athletes or those engaged in regular physical activity. The same nitrates that aid in blood pressure regulation also improve oxygen use within the body. This means that consuming beetroot can enhance physical performance, increase stamina, and reduce the amount of oxygen needed during exercise.

INCORPORATING BEETROOT INTO YOUR DIET.

Getting beetroot's benefits doesn't require drastic changes to your diet. It can be as simple as adding the vegetable to your salads, drinking a glass of beetroot juice, or incorporating it into soups and stews. For those who might find its earthy taste challenging, combining it with sweet or citrus fruits in a smoothie can make it more palatable.

BEETROOT JUICE: A CONCENTRATED DOSE.

Drinking beetroot juice is perhaps the most effective way to enjoy its blood pressure and energy-boosting benefits. Freshly juiced beetroot retains most of its nutrients and active compounds. Drinking a small glass of beetroot juice daily can be a simple yet powerful addition to a heart-healthy diet.

ROASTED OR BOILED: VERSATILE IN COOKING.

Roasting or boiling beetroot brings out its natural sweetness, making it a delicious addition to meals. Roasted beetroot can be a delightful side dish, salad topping, or even a snack. When boiled, it becomes tender and can be pureed for soups or mixed into dishes for added flavor and nutrition.

BEETROOT LEAVES: DON'T DISCARD THEM.

The leaves of the beetroot are just as nutritious as the root. Rich in calcium, iron, and vitamins A and C, they can be cooked similarly to spinach or other leafy greens. Adding them to your diet increases your intake of essential vitamins and minerals.

A WORD OF CAUTION.

While beetroot is generally safe for most people, it's important to consume it in moderation. Excessive consumption can lead to beetroot's most well-known side effect; beeturia, where urine or stools may turn pink or red. This is harmless but can be alarming for those unaware of it.

EMBRACING BEETROOT IN OUR WELLNESS JOURNEY.

Beetroot's hidden benefits for blood pressure and energy enhancement make it a valuable addition to our dietary choices. Its ability to improve cardiovascular health and enhance physical performance is a testament to the power of natural foods in supporting our health. As we continue to uncover the secrets of nature's pantry, beetroot stands out as a bright example of how simple dietary choices can have profound impacts on our well-being.

In our journey towards health and vitality, embracing beetroot is more than just adding a vegetable to our diet; it's about acknowledging and utilizing the gifts of nature in their purest form. It's a step towards harmonizing our health practices with the wisdom of the natural world, a principle that Barbara O'Neill and many advocates of natural health have long encouraged. So, let's raise a glass of beetroot juice to good health, vitality, and the enduring power of nature's goodness.

THE LITTLE-KNOWN HEALTH BENEFITS OF SWEET POTATOES.

Sweet potatoes, with their vibrant color and delicious taste, are not just a culinary delight but also a treasure trove of health benefits. Often overshadowed by their regular potato cousins, these roots possess qualities that might surprise many health enthusiasts. In a delightful blend of traditional wisdom and modern nutrition science, let's uncover the lesser-known health benefits of sweet potatoes, a topic that would surely resonate with natural health advocates like Barbara O'Neill.

A BRIEF HISTORY OF SWEET POTATOES.

Originating in Central and South America, sweet potatoes have been nourished and cherished for thousands of years. Their journey from a staple crop of ancient civilizations to a beloved ingredient in modern kitchens is a testament to their enduring nutritional value and versatility. Barbara O'Neill often emphasizes the significance of such historically rich foods, which are not only packed with nutrients but also with the wisdom of our ancestors.

NUTRITIONAL PROFILE: A POWERHOUSE OF VITAMINS AND MINERALS.

Sweet potatoes are a nutritional powerhouse. They are rich in vitamins, minerals, and antioxidants, each contributing to various aspects of our health. One of their most notable nutrients is beta-carotene, a powerful antioxidant that the body converts into vitamin A, essential for eye health, immune function, and skin health. They are also an excellent source of vitamin C, manganese, copper, and B vitamins.

Regulating Blood Sugar and Supporting Weight Loss.

Contrary to popular belief, sweet potatoes can be beneficial for blood sugar regulation. Their high fiber content helps slow down the release of sugar into the bloodstream, providing a stable energy source and preventing blood sugar spikes. This attribute, combined with their relatively low calorie content, makes them an excellent food choice for weight management and even for diabetic diets, underlining Barbara O'Neill's teachings about the importance of choosing foods that naturally regulate blood sugar.

Heart Health: More Than Just a Tasty Root.

Sweet potatoes also boast heart-healthy properties. The high fiber content aids in reducing cholesterol levels in the blood. They contain potassium, a mineral that helps maintain a healthy balance of fluids and electrolytes and ensures proper heart function.

Digestive Health and Gut Wellbeing.

The dietary fibers in sweet potatoes are not just great for blood sugar and heart health; they also play a crucial role in digestive health. Fiber aids in bowel regularity and prevents constipation. Furthermore, sweet potatoes contain resistant starch, which feeds the beneficial bacteria in our gut, thus contributing to a healthy gut microbiome.

Boosting Immunity and Reducing Inflammation.

The rich color of sweet potatoes indicates their high antioxidant content, particularly beta-carotene and anthocyanins. These antioxidants help in fighting inflammation and boosting the body's immunity. Regular consumption of sweet potatoes can be a natural way to strengthen the body's defense mechanisms against various diseases.

VERSATILITY IN THE KITCHEN.

One of the best things about sweet potatoes is their versatility. They can be baked, boiled, roasted, or mashed. From savory dishes like soups and stews to sweet treats like pies and puddings, sweet potatoes can add nutritional value and flavor to a wide range of recipes. They can also be a healthier alternative to regular potatoes for dishes like fries and wedges.

INCORPORATING SWEET POTATOES INTO YOUR DIET.

Incorporating sweet potatoes into your diet is simple. They can be a side dish, a main course, or even a snack. A baked sweet potato with a sprinkle of cinnamon makes for a delicious and healthy treat, while adding them to salads, soups, and curries can enrich your meals with their unique flavor and health benefits.

A WORD OF CAUTION.

While sweet potatoes are undoubtedly healthy, moderation is key. High in carbohydrates, they should be consumed in a balanced way, especially by those monitoring their carb intake. As with any dietary change, it's important to consider your personal health needs and consult with a healthcare provider if necessary.

A SWEET ADDITION TO YOUR HEALTH JOURNEY.

Sweet potatoes, with their delightful taste and impressive health benefits, are a wonderful addition to a health-conscious diet. Their ability to support various aspects of our health, from blood sugar regulation to boosting immunity, makes them a valuable food choice. Embracing sweet potatoes is about more than just enjoying their flavor; it's about acknowledging and utilizing the gifts of nature in their most wholesome form.

Revitalizing Meals: Quick and Healthy Recipes.

Finding time for nutritious and revitalizing meals can be a challenge in our recent world. Yet, the secret to maintaining vibrant health and energy often lies in our daily diet. Inculcating quick, wholesome recipes can transform our meals from mundane to extraordinary, nourishing our bodies and delighting our palates.

The Philosophy Behind Quick, Nutritious Cooking.

The art of creating quick and healthy meals is about making conscious choices that benefit our health. It includes selecting ingredients that are rich in nutrients, easy to prepare, and naturally flavorful. Barbara O'Neill often speaks about the significance of incorporating a variety of natural, whole foods into our diet to ensure we receive the necessary vitamins, minerals, and antioxidants for optimal health.

Building a Foundation with Whole Foods.

The cornerstone of any revitalizing meal is whole, unprocessed foods. These include fresh fruits and vegetables, whole grains, lean proteins, and healthy fats. By building our meals around these components, we can ensure that each dish is not only quick to prepare but also packed with nutritional benefits.

Revitalizing Breakfasts to Start Your Day.

A nutritious breakfast sets the tone for the day. Here are a couple of quick and healthy breakfast ideas:

- Overnight Oats: Mix rolled oats with your choice of milk or yogurt, add a spoonful of chia seeds for extra fiber, and let it sit overnight. In the morning, top it with fresh fruits and nuts.

- Smoothie Bowls: Blend your favorite fruits with a bit of spinach or kale for an extra nutrient kick. Pour it into a bowl and top with sliced fruits, seeds, and a drizzle of honey.

ENERGIZING LUNCHES FOR BUSY DAYS.

Lunches should be light yet fulfilling to keep you energized throughout the day. Some quick options include:

- Quinoa Salad: Cook quinoa and let it cool. Mix it with chopped vegetables, a handful of greens, and your favorite dressing.

- Wraps: Use whole grain wraps to roll up a combination of lean protein (like grilled chicken or tofu), lots of fresh veggies, and a spread like hummus or avocado.

DINNERS THAT NOURISH AND SATISFY.

Dinner is a time to unwind and nourish your body with a hearty meal. Some simple, healthy dinner ideas are:

- Stir-Fry: Quickly stir-fry a variety of vegetables and a protein source like shrimp or tempeh. Serve it over brown rice or quinoa.

- Soup: Prepare a vegetable or lentil soup with broth, mixed vegetables, and seasonings. Soups are comforting and can be made in large batches for convenience.

Snacks: Quick, Healthy Options.

Healthy snacks are crucial for keeping energy levels up between meals. Opt for fruits, nuts, yogurt, or homemade granola bars. These snacks provide a quick energy boost without the sugar crash associated with processed snacks.

Hydration: An Essential Component.

Alongside these meals, don't forget the importance of hydration. Herbal teas, infused water, and natural juices are excellent for keeping you hydrated and can be a refreshing complement to your meals.

The Role of Herbs and Spices.

Herbs and spices not only add flavor without extra calories but also offer various health benefits. Incorporate herbs like basil, parsley, or cilantro, and spices like turmeric, ginger, and cinnamon into your recipes to enhance both taste and nutritional value.

Meal Prepping: A Time-Saving Strategy.

One of Barbara O'Neill's teachings is about being proactive in our health choices, and meal prepping aligns perfectly with this philosophy. By dedicating a few hours each week to preparing ingredients or entire meals, you can save time and ensure that you always have healthy options on hand.

Celebrating the Joy of Healthy Eating.

Creating quick and healthy meals is an enjoyable and rewarding experience. It's about celebrating the natural flavors of whole foods, being creative in the kitchen, and making choices that support our health and well-being. In a world where we often find ourselves short on time, these quick and revitalizing recipes offer a way to maintain a healthy diet without compromising on taste or nutrition.

Each meal is an opportunity to nourish your body, delight your senses, and embrace a healthier lifestyle. So, let's cherish the joy of cooking and the pleasure of eating, knowing that with each dish, we are taking steps toward a more vibrant, healthier life.

Baking Soda Wonders: From Cleaning to Health.

Baking soda, a humble kitchen staple, often relegated to the back of the pantry, holds a plethora of uses that extend far beyond baking. This unassuming white powder is a powerhouse of versatility, offering benefits in cleaning, health, and beauty that many might find surprising.

A Brief History of Baking Soda.

Baking soda, or sodium bicarbonate, has been used for centuries. Originating as a natural compound, it has been utilized in various cultures for baking, cleaning, and even medicinal purposes. Its rise in popularity is a testament to its effectiveness and safety, qualities that are often highlighted in Barbara O'Neill's teachings about using natural substances for health and home.

Baking Soda in the Home: A Natural Cleaning Agent.

One of the most well-known uses of baking soda is as a cleaning agent. Its mildly abrasive texture and natural deodorizing properties make it an excellent choice for a variety of household chores.

- Surface Cleaner: A paste made from baking soda and water can clean and deodorize kitchen counters, stainless steel sinks, and even cooking utensils.

- Carpet Freshener: Sprinkling baking soda on carpets, letting it sit, and then vacuuming it up can help remove odors and freshen the room.

- Natural Deodorizer: Placing a box of baking soda in the refrigerator or mixing it with essential oils for a room deodorizer are simple ways to keep your home smelling fresh without the use of chemicals.

BAKING SODA FOR PERSONAL CARE: BEYOND BEAUTY.

Baking soda's utility extends to personal care, where it can be used in several ways:

- Toothpaste and Oral Health: Its mild abrasive properties make baking soda an effective tooth cleaner. Mixed with a bit of water, it can serve as a simple, natural toothpaste, promoting oral hygiene and whiter teeth.

- Skin Care: A gentle exfoliant for the skin, baking soda can be used in homemade facial scrubs to remove dead skin cells without harsh chemicals.

- Hair Care: Some people use baking soda as a natural shampoo alternative. It can help remove buildup from commercial hair products, leaving the hair clean and refreshed.

BAKING SODA IN HEALTH REMEDIES.

In addition to its cleaning and beauty applications, baking soda has several health-related uses:

- Indigestion and Heartburn Relief: Baking soda can neutralize stomach acid, making it a quick and effective remedy for indigestion and heartburn.

- Soothing Baths: Adding baking soda to a bath can help soothe irritated skin, relieve itching, and soften the skin.

- Foot Care: A baking soda foot soak can help relieve foot odor and soften rough skin.

IN THE KITCHEN: BEYOND BAKING.

While its primary use is in baking, baking soda also has other culinary applications:

- Natural Leavening Agent: It's a key ingredient in many baked goods, helping them to rise and achieve the desired texture.

- Vegetable Cleaning: Baking soda can be used to clean fruits and vegetables, helping to remove dirt and residue.

BAKING SODA FOR GARDENING.

Gardeners will find baking soda helpful in their pursuit of natural gardening:

- Pest Control: A natural pest deterrent, it can be used to keep away certain insects and pests without the need for harsh chemicals.

- Plant Care: Baking soda can be used to treat fungal growth on plants, keeping them healthy and thriving.

A CAUTIONARY NOTE.

While baking soda is safe and versatile, it's important to use it correctly. Its alkaline nature means it should be used judiciously, especially when it comes to personal care. Overuse on the skin or hair might lead to dryness. Additionally, when ingested for health purposes, it should be done so in moderation and not as a substitute for medical treatment.

EMBRACING THE WONDERS OF BAKING SODA.

Baking soda's multitude of uses, from cleaning and deodorizing to health and beauty, makes it a must-have in every home. Its simplicity, effectiveness, and safety align with the teachings of Barbara O'Neill, who advocate for the use of natural, non-toxic substances in our daily lives. As we look forward to a healthier, more sustainable lifestyle, baking soda stands as a shining example of how everyday items can have extraordinary uses.

SNACKS AND BEVERAGES: EASY AND NUTRITIOUS OPTIONS.

Snacks and beverages can play a pivotal role in our health and wellness. They are not just stop-gaps between meals but can be moments of nourishment and enjoyment. In line with Barbara O'Neill's teachings, which emphasize natural, wholesome foods, let's find out how snacks and drinks can be both delightful and beneficial.

THE PHILOSOPHY BEHIND NUTRITIOUS SNACKING AND SIPPING.

Nutritious snacking is more than choosing healthy foods; it's about understanding the body's needs and responding with nourishment. Healthy snacks can provide energy boosts, essential nutrients, and even help maintain a healthy weight. Similarly, choosing the right beverages can aid hydration, provide nutrients, and offer health benefits.

SNACKING WITH A PURPOSE.

The key to healthy snacking is intentionality; choosing snacks that are both satisfying and nutritious. A well-chosen snack can curb hunger, provide a boost of energy, and prevent overeating at meal times.

- Nuts and Seeds: A handful of mixed nuts or seeds is a quick, nutrient-dense snack. They are rich in healthy fats, proteins, and fiber, making them an excellent choice for a satisfying snack.

- Fresh Fruits and Vegetables: Nature's fast food, fruits, and vegetables, provide vitamins, minerals, and fiber.

45

Pairing them with dips like hummus or nut butter can make them even more enjoyable.

CREATIVE SNACK IDEAS.

Getting creative with your snacks can make them more appealing and fun to eat:

- Fruit Kebabs: Skewer pieces of your favorite fruits for a fun and colorful snack.

- Vegetable Chips: Kale, sweet potato, or beet chips baked with a sprinkle of salt can be a healthy alternative to store-bought chips.

- Energy Balls: Combine oats, nuts, seeds, and dried fruits in a food processor, roll into balls, and enjoy a homemade energy booster.

BEVERAGES FOR HYDRATION AND HEALTH.

Drinking the right beverages is just as important as eating the right foods. Water is essential, but other drinks can also contribute to our daily nutrient intake.

- Herbal Teas: A soothing cup of herbal tea can provide antioxidants and hydration without the caffeine found in regular tea or coffee.

- Fruit Infused Water: Infusing water with fruits like lemon, berries, or cucumber adds flavor without added sugar.

HEALTHY BEVERAGE OPTIONS.

Beyond water and herbal teas, there are other beverages that can be both nutritious and refreshing:

- Green Smoothies: Blend leafy greens like spinach or kale with fruits for a nutrient-packed drink.

- Nut Milk: Almond, coconut, or oat milk can be a nutritious, dairy-free beverage option.

THE ROLE OF BEVERAGES IN A BALANCED DIET.

Beverages can play an important role in a balanced diet. They can help in detoxification, digestion, and even weight management. For instance, green tea is known for its metabolism-boosting properties.

SNACK AND BEVERAGE PREPPING.

To ensure you always have healthy options on hand, snack and beverage prepping can be a lifesaver. Preparing portions of nuts, chopping fruits and vegetables, or making a batch of healthy drinks at the start of the week can make nutritious snacking more convenient.

LISTENING TO YOUR BODY.

One of Barbara O'Neill's teachings is to listen to your body. This is crucial when it comes to snacking and drinking. Understanding your body's hunger and thirst signals, and differentiating them from emotional eating, is key to mindful consumption.

THE JOY OF HEALTHY SNACKING AND SIPPING.

Incorporating nutritious snacks and beverages into your daily routine is an easy and delicious way to enhance your overall health. These mini-meals and drinks can provide essential nutrients, boost energy, and even contribute to a healthy lifestyle. In our busy lives, these quick and nutritious options are not just conveniences; they are small, yet powerful, affirmations of our commitment to health and well-being.

CREATING POSITIVE ENERGY AT HOME: BAY LEAVES AND GARLIC USES.

The use of natural elements to create a positive atmosphere is a timeless practice. Among these natural allies, bay leaves and garlic stand out, not only for their culinary uses but also for their lesser-known ability to enhance the energy of our living spaces. This exposition into the uses of bay leaves and garlic at home blends traditional wisdom with a touch of modern understanding, embodying the nurturing and holistic approach to life.

BAY LEAVES: MORE THAN JUST A CULINARY HERB.

Bay leaves, known for their robust flavor in cooking, have a history steeped in folklore and traditional practices. In ancient times, they were associated with protection and purification, used in rituals to ward off negativity. Today, their subtle, woodsy aroma continues to be valued, not just in the kitchen, but also as a tool for creating a serene and positive home environment.

- Bay Leaves for Energy Cleansing: Burning bay leaves is an age-old practice for energy cleansing. The smoke from burning bay leaves is believed to purify the air and dispel negative energy. To practice this, simply light a dried bay leaf and allow the smoke to waft through your home, paying special attention to corners and doorways where stagnant energy might gather.

- A Natural Insect Repellent: Bay leaves are a natural deterrent for pests like cockroaches, moths, and ants. Placing dried bay leaves in cupboards, drawers, and pantry areas can help keep these unwanted visitors at bay.

- Stress Relief and Relaxation: The aroma of bay leaves has a calming effect on the mind and body. Boiling bay leaves in water and allowing the scent to permeate your home can create a tranquil atmosphere, aiding in stress relief and relaxation.

GARLIC: A POTENT PROTECTOR IN FOLKLORE AND HEALTH.

Garlic, much revered in the culinary world, also holds a place of significance in folklore and traditional healing practices. It has been used throughout history as a symbol of protection and a ward against negative influences.

- Garlic for Purifying Spaces: Similar to bay leaves, garlic is believed to possess protective qualities. Hanging garlic cloves in entryways or windows is an old practice thought to guard against negative energy entering the home.

- Health Benefits in the Home: Beyond its protective lore, garlic is renowned for its health benefits, which Barbara O'Neill often highlights. It's a natural antibacterial and antiviral agent, making it a valuable ally during cold and flu season. Including garlic in your daily diet can boost your immune system and improve overall health.

- Natural Pest Control: Garlic's strong scent is also effective in repelling pests. Planting garlic in your garden can help protect other plants, and placing garlic cloves near areas where pests are a problem can be a natural way to control them.

INCORPORATING BAY LEAVES AND GARLIC INTO DAILY LIFE.

Bringing bay leaves and garlic into your daily routine can be simple and enjoyable:

- Cooking with Bay Leaves and Garlic: Incorporate these ingredients into your cooking for both their flavor and health benefits. They can be added to soups, stews, and sauces, infusing dishes with depth and nutrition.

- DIY Home Fragrances: Create natural home fragrances with bay leaves and garlic. Simmering water with bay leaves, garlic, and other aromatic herbs can fill your home with a comforting and cleansing aroma.

- Homemade Health Remedies: Utilize garlic in homemade remedies for its health-boosting properties. Garlic-infused oils or teas can be effective in treating minor ailments and boosting immunity.

A NOTE OF CAUTION.

While using bay leaves and garlic in the home is generally safe, it's important to practice caution. Burning bay leaves should be done carefully and in a well-ventilated area. Additionally, those with specific allergies should be mindful when handling these ingredients.

EMBRACING NATURE'S GIFTS FOR A HARMONIOUS HOME.

The use of bay leaves and garlic for creating positive energy at home is a beautiful example of how nature's gifts can be utilized in our daily lives. These practices, grounded in tradition and supported by modern understanding, offer a natural, holistic way to enhance our living spaces. They remind us of the simplicity and effectiveness of natural solutions and encourage us to embrace these gentle yet powerful tools in our quest for a harmonious, healthy home.

Refreshing Lemon and Egg Wellness Recipes.

Lemons and eggs emerge as two versatile heroes in recent years. While each is commonly found in kitchens worldwide, their combination in wellness recipes can be both refreshing and beneficial. In this article, we expose the effective ways to incorporate these everyday ingredients into your wellness routine.

Lemons: A Burst of Vitamin C and More.

Lemons, with their zesty flavor and high vitamin C content, have long been revered for their health benefits. They aid in digestion, boost the immune system, and promote healthy skin. But their usefulness extends far beyond these commonly known benefits.

- Detoxification: Lemons are known for their detoxifying properties. Starting your day with a glass of warm lemon water can kick-start your digestive system and help flush out toxins.

- Skin Care: The antioxidants in lemons can help fight skin aging. A simple face mask made from lemon juice and egg whites can tighten pores and brighten the skin.

Eggs: Nutritional Powerhouses.

Eggs are a staple in many diets, valued for their high-quality protein and range of vitamins and minerals. They're particularly rich in B vitamins, essential for energy production, and eye health.

- Hair Care: The proteins and nutrients in eggs can nourish hair. An egg mask, when applied to hair, can strengthen, add shine, and promote hair growth.

- Healthy Breakfasts: Eggs are incredibly versatile for cooking. They can be the centerpiece of a nutritious, filling breakfast, providing sustained energy throughout the day.

COMBINING LEMONS AND EGGS IN WELLNESS RECIPES.

The combination of lemons and eggs might seem unusual, but together, they can create refreshing and healthful recipes. Let's explore some simple yet effective recipes that harness their combined benefits.

- Lemon and Egg Face Mask for Skin Care: Beat an egg white until frothy and mix in a few drops of lemon juice. Apply the mixture to your face, leave it on for 10-15 minutes, and then rinse off. This mask can help reduce oiliness, tighten pores, and give your skin a fresh glow.

- Egg Lemonade for a Post-Workout Drink: After a strenuous workout, try a protein-rich lemonade. Mix freshly squeezed lemon juice, a teaspoon of honey, a pinch of salt, and a raw egg in a glass of water. This drink can provide hydration, protein, and a quick energy boost.

INCORPORATING LEMONS AND EGGS INTO DAILY WELLNESS.

To make the most of lemons and eggs in your daily routine, consider the following tips:

- Morning Ritual with Lemon Water: Start your day with a glass of warm lemon water to hydrate and activate your digestive system.

- Egg-Based Breakfasts: Incorporate eggs into your breakfast for a nutritious start to the day. Pair them with vegetables for an even healthier meal.

- Lemon in Salads and Meals: Use lemon juice in salads, as a dressing, or to add flavor to cooked meals. Its acidity can enhance the taste and increase the absorption of iron from your foods.

CAUTIONS AND CONSIDERATIONS.

While lemons and eggs are generally safe for most people, there are a few considerations to keep in mind:

- Raw Eggs: Consuming raw eggs carries a risk of Salmonella infection. It's important to use fresh, properly stored eggs if you choose to consume them raw.

- Lemon and Skin Sensitivity: Lemon juice can make the skin more sensitive to sunlight. After using lemon on your skin, it's advisable to avoid direct sun exposure and use sunscreen.

CELEBRATING SIMPLICITY IN WELLNESS.

The use of lemons and eggs in wellness recipes is a delightful celebration of simplicity and natural health. These recipes showcase how everyday ingredients can be transformed into tools for enhancing our well-being. Whether it's through a nourishing breakfast, a revitalizing drink, or a natural skin care treatment, lemons and eggs offer an array of benefits that are easy to incorporate into our daily routines.

Zucchini's Secret: Regulating Blood Sugar Naturally.

Often relegated to the role of a simple side dish, this unassuming vegetable harbors a secret superpower: its ability to help regulate blood sugar naturally. Let's take a look at how zucchini can be a delightful and effective ally in maintaining healthy blood sugar levels.

Unveiling Zucchini's Nutritional Profile.

Zucchini, also known as courgette, is a summer squash that belongs to the Cucurbitaceae plant family. It's not only low in calories but also high in essential nutrients, making it an excellent addition to a health-conscious diet. Rich in dietary fiber, antioxidants, and essential vitamins like B6, K, and C, zucchini supports various aspects of health, including blood sugar regulation.

The Role of Fiber in Blood Sugar Control.

One of zucchini's standout features is its high fiber content. Fiber plays a crucial role in stabilizing blood sugar levels by slowing down the absorption of sugar into the bloodstream. This helps prevent the sharp spikes in blood sugar that can occur after eating. Including zucchini in your meals can therefore contribute to more balanced and stable blood sugar levels throughout the day.

Zucchini and Type 2 Diabetes Management.

For individuals managing type 2 diabetes, incorporating zucchini into the diet can be particularly beneficial. The low carbohydrate content and glycemic index of zucchini make it an ideal food for maintaining healthy blood sugar levels. Additionally, the antioxidants present in zucchini, such as lutein and zeaxanthin, offer protective benefits against the complications associated with diabetes.

VERSATILE AND DELICIOUS: INCORPORATING ZUCCHINI INTO YOUR DIET.

Zucchini's versatility in the kitchen makes it easy to incorporate into your daily diet. Here are some delightful ways to enjoy zucchini:

- Zucchini Noodles: A healthy alternative to traditional pasta, zucchini noodles can be topped with your favorite sauce for a nutritious, low-carb meal.

- Grilled or Roasted Zucchini: Simply slice and grill or roast with a bit of olive oil, salt, and pepper for a simple yet delicious side dish.

- Zucchini Soup: Blend cooked zucchini with herbs and broth to create a soothing and nutritious soup.

REFRESHING ZUCCHINI RECIPES FOR BLOOD SUGAR MANAGEMENT.

Let's look into some specific recipes that not only taste good but also contribute to blood sugar regulation:

- Zucchini and Basil Salad: Combine thinly sliced zucchini with fresh basil, a sprinkle of lemon juice, and a dash of olive oil for a refreshing salad.

- Stuffed Zucchini Boats: Hollow out zucchini halves and fill them with a mixture of lean ground meat, vegetables, and herbs, then bake until tender.

Zucchini's Hydration Benefits.

Besides its direct impact on blood sugar, zucchini is also high in water content, promoting hydration. Proper hydration is essential for overall health and can indirectly support blood sugar regulation by aiding in metabolic processes.

A Note on Portion Sizes and Preparation.

While zucchini is beneficial for blood sugar control, it's important to consider portion sizes and preparation methods. Overconsumption of any food, even vegetables like zucchini, can lead to imbalances, and cooking methods that add excessive calories or unhealthy fats can negate the vegetable's natural health benefits.

Embracing Zucchini in a Balanced Diet.

Zucchini's ability to help regulate blood sugar is a wonderful example of how everyday vegetables can play a significant role in our health. Its versatility, flavor, and nutritional profile make it an ideal ingredient for anyone looking to maintain or improve their blood sugar levels naturally. Let's utilize zucchini's hidden powers, making it a regular, delightful presence in our meals and our journey towards balanced health.

Salt and Toothpaste: Unusual Health Benefits.

Salt and toothpaste are two humble yet potent allies. Far beyond their basic uses in seasoning food and cleaning teeth, these common household staples possess a range of unusual health benefits that align with the principles of natural healing. Drawing inspiration from natural health advocates like Barbara O'Neill, let's get into the uses of salt and toothpaste, getting to see their lesser-known roles in promoting health and wellness.

The Healing Wonders of Salt.

Salt, particularly unrefined sea salt or Himalayan pink salt, has been valued for centuries, not only for its flavor-enhancing properties but also for its therapeutic qualities. Rich in minerals, salt can play a crucial role in various home remedies.

- Soothing Sore Throats: Gargling with warm salt water is a time-honored remedy for soothing sore throats. The salt helps reduce swelling and discomfort by drawing out fluids from the throat tissues.

- Natural Oral Health Care: Salt can be used as a gentle tooth polisher and breath freshener. Mixing salt with water can create a simple yet effective mouth rinse that helps in neutralizing bad breath and cleansing the oral cavity.

- Detox Baths: Adding salt to your bath water can create a detoxifying and relaxing experience. The minerals in the salt can help soothe muscles, reduce stress, and promote skin health.

Toothpaste: Beyond Brightening Smiles.

With its gentle abrasive and cleansing properties, toothpaste can be repurposed in several health and beauty applications.

- Relieving Minor Burns and Insect Bites: Applying a small amount of toothpaste to a minor burn or insect bite can provide relief. The cooling properties of toothpaste help soothe the skin and reduce itching and irritation.

- Enhancing Skin Care: Toothpaste can be used as a spot treatment for pimples. Its ingredients can help dry out the pimple and reduce its appearance.

- Polishing and Cleaning: Toothpaste can be used to clean and polish various items, from jewelry to iron surfaces. Its mild abrasive quality makes it effective in removing tarnish and stains.

Combining Salt and Toothpaste: A Dynamic Duo.

When combined, salt and toothpaste can create powerful concoctions for health and beauty purposes:

- Homemade Scrubs: Mixing salt with toothpaste creates a homemade scrub that can be used for exfoliating the skin or even for smoothing rough areas like elbows and heels.

- Enhanced Oral Care: Adding a pinch of salt to toothpaste can boost its effectiveness in removing plaque and stains from teeth, leading to brighter and cleaner teeth.

CREATIVE AND PRACTICAL USES IN DAILY LIFE.

Expanding the use of salt and toothpaste into your daily routine can be both creative and practical. Here are some ideas:

- Salt as a Natural Deodorizer: Placing a bowl of salt in the refrigerator or a room can help absorb odors and freshen the air.

- Toothpaste for Clearing Foggy Mirrors: Rubbing a small amount of toothpaste on bathroom mirrors can prevent them from fogging up during showers.

HEALTH PRECAUTIONS AND BEST PRACTICES.

While salt and toothpaste offer various benefits, it's essential to use them wisely:

- Be Mindful of Salt Intake: Excessive salt consumption can lead to health issues. When using salt for health remedies, moderation is key.

- Choose the Right Toothpaste: For non-dental uses, it's best to use plain white toothpaste without added whitening agents or microgranules.

EMBRACING THE UNCONVENTIONAL.

The unconventional uses of salt and toothpaste are shining examples of how everyday items can be reimagined for health and wellness. These simple yet effective remedies and hacks not only offer practical solutions but also resonate with the ethos of natural living and resourcefulness. When next you reach for the salt shaker or the tube of toothpaste, remember that you're holding more than just culinary or hygiene essentials; you're holding tools for a healthier, more harmonious life.

WELLNESS INSIGHTS: UNUSUAL HEALTH INDICATORS.

The body often communicates through signals and symptoms that might not be immediately apparent. Beyond the usual indicators like pulse rate and body temperature, there are unusual, often overlooked signs that can provide profound insights into our overall health. Let's discuss the less conventional health indicators, offering a blend of traditional wisdom and modern understanding.

1. Nail Health: Windows to Your Internal Well-being.

One often-overlooked indicator of health is the condition of our nails. Brittle, discolored, or ridged nails can be signs of nutritional deficiencies, such as a lack of iron or zinc. White spots on nails, often attributed to calcium deficiency, can also indicate a lack of zinc. Observing changes in nail health can be a subtle yet telling way to monitor internal health.

2. Tongue Appearance: The Mirror of Digestive Health.

In traditional Chinese medicine, the tongue is viewed as a map of internal health, particularly digestive health. A tongue with a thick white coat could indicate an imbalance in gut flora or digestive issues, while a tongue with a bright red tip might signal emotional stress or anxiety.

3. Eye Whites: Indicators of Liver Health.

The color of the whites of your eyes can reveal a lot about your liver health. A yellow tinge may indicate jaundice, often associated with liver dysfunction. Ensuring your diet is rich in liver-supportive nutrients, such as those found in leafy greens, can help maintain liver health and, by extension, clear, bright eye whites.

4. Earlobe Creases: A Surprising Sign.

An unusual but notable indicator is the presence of a crease on the earlobe, often referred to as Frank's sign. Some studies suggest that this crease may be linked to an increased risk of heart disease and should prompt a more thorough cardiovascular health assessment.

5. Sleep Patterns: More Than Just Rest.

Your sleep patterns can also be a significant indicator of health. Difficulty falling asleep or staying asleep can be signs of stress, anxiety, or hormonal imbalances. On the other hand, consistently feeling refreshed and energized upon waking is a good sign of both physical and mental well-being.

6. Body Odor: A Reflection of Metabolic Changes.

Changes in body odor can reflect various metabolic changes. For instance, a sudden change in the way your sweat smells could be a sign of changes in diet, hormonal imbalances, or even infections. Paying attention to these changes can provide early clues to internal health changes.

7. Scalp Condition: More Than Skin Deep.

The health of your scalp can reflect the state of your internal health. A dry, itchy scalp can indicate a deficiency in essential fatty acids, while an excessively oily scalp could signal hormonal imbalances.

8. Frequency of Sighing: A Clue to Emotional Health.

An increase in the frequency of sighs can be a subtle indicator of emotional health, often pointing to increased stress or emotional distress. Observing these changes can prompt you to take steps to manage stress, such as practicing mindfulness or seeking emotional support.

9. Skin Elasticity: A Sign of Hydration and Aging.

The skin's elasticity, often checked by the 'pinch test' (pinching the skin on the back of the hand and seeing how quickly it returns to its original state), can indicate hydration levels and skin aging. Decreased elasticity might suggest the need for better hydration or increased antioxidant intake to combat skin aging.

10. Menstrual Cycle Regularity: A Gauge of Hormonal Balance.

For women, the regularity and nature of the menstrual cycle can be a significant indicator of hormonal health. Irregularities in the cycle can be signs of conditions like polycystic ovary syndrome (PCOS) or thyroid imbalances.

EMBRACING A HOLISTIC VIEW OF HEALTH.

Understanding these unusual health indicators requires a holistic view of health, one that encompasses physical, emotional, and mental well-being. By paying attention to these less conventional signs, we can gain a deeper understanding of our health and take proactive steps to maintain it.

NATURAL COLD AND FLU REMEDIES: GINGER AND LEMON.

Ginger and lemon stand out as two venerable allies in the battle against cold and flu. These humble kitchen staples, revered in traditional medicine and validated by modern science, are more than just ingredients for a comforting tea; they are nature's gift in bolstering our defenses against seasonal ailments. Inspired by the teachings of natural health advocates like Barbara O'Neill, let's see the delightful synergy of ginger and lemon in combating cold and flu, blending their traditional uses with contemporary insights.

GINGER: THE WARMING WONDER ROOT.

Ginger, with its pungent flavor and warming properties, has been a cornerstone in herbal medicine for centuries. Its active component, gingerol, is responsible for its potent anti-inflammatory and antioxidant effects.

- Combatting Nausea and Digestive Discomfort: Ginger is renowned for its ability to soothe nausea, making it a go-to remedy for flu-related stomach upset. It also aids in digestion, ensuring that the body's energy is focused on fighting off infections rather than dealing with digestive distress.

- Enhancing Immune Response: Ginger's anti-inflammatory properties help in reducing the symptoms of a sore throat, a common precursor to colds and flu. Its warming effect also promotes sweating, which can be beneficial in lowering fevers associated with the flu.

LEMON: A CITRUSY BOOST OF VITAMIN C.

Lemon, the bright and zesty citrus fruit, is not just a flavor enhancer. It's packed with vitamin C, a crucial nutrient for immune function.

- Strengthening Immunity: Vitamin C in lemons contributes to immune defense by supporting various cellular functions of the body's immune system. It's particularly beneficial in preventing and treating respiratory infections.

- Detoxifying the Body: Lemon aids in detoxification, an essential process during illness, by stimulating the liver and enhancing the body's ability to purge toxins.

Creating Healing Concoctions with Ginger and Lemon.

The combination of ginger and lemon creates a potent remedy for cold and flu symptoms. Here are some delightful ways to harness their powers:

- Ginger-Lemon Tea: Boil sliced ginger in water and add fresh lemon juice. This simple tea can be consumed several times a day to relieve symptoms of cold and flu.

- Honey, Ginger, and Lemon Syrup: Combine equal parts of honey, ginger juice, and lemon juice. This syrup can be taken as is or added to tea for a soothing remedy.

GINGER AND LEMON IN DAILY HEALTH ROUTINES.

Incorporating ginger and lemon into your daily routine, especially during cold and flu season, can bolster your immune system:

- Start Your Day with Lemon Water: A glass of warm water with lemon juice in the morning can kickstart your digestive system and boost your immunity.

- Add Ginger to Meals: Grate fresh ginger into soups, stews, or stir-fries to enhance flavor and reap its health benefits.

LIFESTYLE TIPS TO COMPLEMENT GINGER AND LEMON REMEDIES.

To maximize the effectiveness of ginger and lemon in fighting colds and flu, consider these lifestyle tips:

- Stay Hydrated: Fluids are crucial when fighting off infections. Ensure you're drinking plenty of water alongside your ginger and lemon remedies.

- Rest and Relaxation: Allow your body to heal by getting enough rest. Sleep is a critical component of a strong immune response.

PRECAUTIONS AND CONSIDERATIONS.

While ginger and lemon are generally safe, some precautions should be taken:

- Ginger and Blood Thinning: Ginger has blood-thinning properties. If you are on blood-thinning medication, consult with a healthcare provider before consuming large amounts of ginger.

- Acidity of Lemon: Be mindful of the acidity in lemon, especially if you have a sensitive stomach or acid reflux.

Embracing Nature's Simplicity in Healing.

The use of ginger and lemon in combating colds and flu is a beautiful illustration of nature's simplicity and effectiveness in healing. These remedies, steeped in tradition yet supported by scientific research, offer a comforting, natural way to alleviate symptoms and boost overall health.

THE NUTRITIONAL POWER OF BEETS.

Nestled in the heart of the vegetable garden, beets quietly radiate their deep, earthy charm. Often overlooked for more flashy vegetables, beets possess a nutritional prowess that can play a vital role in maintaining health and vitality. With their rich, vibrant color and a host of health benefits, beets are a treasure trove of goodness. Let's unearth the myriad ways in which this humble root vegetable can enhance our wellness, blending traditional wisdom with modern nutritional insights.

BEETS: A HISTORICAL SUPERFOOD.

Beets have been nourishing humanity since ancient times. Originally, it was their leaves that were consumed, while the sweet red root that we enjoy today was developed over time. This evolution marks beets as a food deeply intertwined with human history, offering both sustenance and medicinal benefits.

NUTRITIONAL PROFILE: WHAT MAKES BEETS A SUPERFOOD.

Beets are nutritional powerhouses. They are low in calories yet high in valuable vitamins and minerals. In particular, beets are rich in folate, manganese, potassium, iron, and vitamin C. They are also a fantastic source of dietary nitrates, which have a profound effect on heart health and blood pressure.

1. Heart Health and Blood Pressure.

The nitrates in beets are converted into nitric oxide in the body, which helps to relax and dilate blood vessels, improving blood flow and lowering blood pressure. This makes beets an excellent food for heart health. Regular consumption of beetroot juice has been shown to have a significant effect on controlling blood pressure.

2. Athletic Performance Enhancement.

For those looking to boost their athletic performance, beets might just be the secret ingredient. The nitrates in beets improve the efficiency of mitochondria, the energy-producing cells in our bodies, which can enhance stamina and endurance.

3. Anti-Inflammatory and Detoxification Properties.

Beets contain betalains, pigments that give them their red color and possess strong anti-inflammatory properties. These compounds can help protect against certain chronic diseases and are also beneficial for detoxification, aiding in purging toxins from the body.

4. Digestive Health.

High in fiber, beets support digestive health by preventing constipation and promoting regularity for a healthy digestive tract. They are also beneficial for gut health, as their fiber content feeds beneficial gut bacteria.

5. Cognitive Function.

The nitrates in beets can also boost cognitive function. By increasing blood flow to the brain, beets may help improve mental and cognitive functions, especially in older adults.

INCORPORATING BEETS INTO YOUR DIET.

There are many delicious and simple ways to add beets to your diet:

- Roasted Beets: Roasting beets brings out their natural sweetness. Simply toss them with a bit of olive oil and roast until tender.

- Beetroot Juice: A popular way to enjoy beets, beetroot juice can be a refreshing and potent drink, especially before workouts.

- Beet Salads: Grated raw beets make a crunchy, nutritious addition to salads.

- Beet Greens: Don't discard the leafy green tops of beets! They can be cooked and enjoyed in the same way as spinach.

COMBINING BEETS WITH OTHER SUPERFOODS.

To maximize the health benefits, combine beets with other superfoods. For example, a salad with beets, nuts, and leafy greens is not only nutritionally dense but also a delight for the taste buds.

BEET RECIPES FOR WELLNESS.

Here are a couple of simple recipes to help you incorporate beets into your diet:

- Beet and Ginger Smoothie: Blend cooked beets, ginger, apple, and a bit of lemon juice for a zesty, health-boosting smoothie.

- Beetroot Hummus: Add cooked beets to your traditional hummus recipe for an extra kick of nutrition and a beautiful color.

A NOTE OF CAUTION.

While beets are incredibly healthy, they should be consumed in moderation. Their high oxalate content can contribute to kidney stones in susceptible individuals.

REDISCOVERING THE HUMBLE BEET.

In rediscovering the humble beet, we reconnect with a part of our ancestral diet that is both nourishing and healing. Beets, with their deep colors and sweet, earthy flavors, remind us that nature's gifts are often simple yet profoundly effective. By incorporating beets into our regular diet, we embrace a food that is not only delicious but also a powerful ally in our quest for health and wellness. So, let's celebrate and savor the beet, a vegetable that truly embodies the richness and wisdom of the natural world.

HOMEMADE MOZZARELLA: HEALTHY AND SIMPLE.

Known for its soft texture and mild, creamy flavor, mozzarella is a favorite in many kitchens. But beyond its culinary appeal lies the joy and health benefits of making mozzarella at home. Let's search the simple art of making homemade mozzarella and how it can be a healthy, enjoyable addition to your culinary skills.

THE ORIGINS OF MOZZARELLA.

Mozzarella originated in Italy, with its roots in the pastoral traditions of the country. Traditionally made from the milk of water buffalos, it has now become popular worldwide and is often made with cow's milk. The process of making mozzarella involves an interesting play of science and art, resulting in a cheese that is not only delicious but also versatile.

NUTRITIONAL BENEFITS OF HOMEMADE MOZZARELLA.

Homemade mozzarella is not just a culinary delight; it's also packed with nutritional benefits. Rich in calcium, protein, and essential vitamins, it contributes to bone health, muscle repair, and overall well-being. By making mozzarella at home, you can also ensure it's free from preservatives and artificial additives often found in commercial varieties.

THE SIMPLE JOY OF MAKING MOZZARELLA AT HOME.

Making mozzarella at home is simpler than you might think. It involves a process known as acidification, followed by coagulation, curd processing, and stretching. The beauty of making mozzarella at home lies in the control it gives you over the ingredients and the process, allowing you to create a cheese that suits your taste and health preferences.

INGREDIENTS AND EQUIPMENT NEEDED.

To make homemade mozzarella, you'll need a few basic ingredients and tools:

- Milk: The star ingredient. Use fresh, high-quality milk for the best results. Traditionally, buffalo milk is used, but cow's milk works well too.

- Citric Acid and Rennet: These are coagulants that help in curdling the milk.

- Salt: For flavor enhancement.

- A Thermometer, a Slotted Spoon, and a Pot: Essential tools for the cheese-making process.

THE PROCESS OF MAKING MOZZARELLA.

- Acidification: Dissolve citric acid in water and add it to the milk. This step prepares the milk for coagulation.

- Coagulation: Heat the milk and add rennet, which helps the milk to coagulate and form curds.

- Curd Processing: Once the curd has formed, cut it and cook it until it reaches the right consistency.

- Stretching: The most fun part! Stretch the curd to achieve mozzarella's signature texture.

CREATIVE WAYS TO ENJOY YOUR HOMEMADE MOZZARELLA.

Once your mozzarella is ready, the possibilities for enjoyment are endless:

- Fresh Caprese Salad: Combine slices of fresh mozzarella with tomatoes, basil, olive oil, salt, and pepper.

- Homemade Pizza: Top your pizza with slices of fresh mozzarella for a delicious, gooey experience.

- Mozzarella Sticks: Coat slices of mozzarella in breadcrumbs and herbs, and bake or fry them for a crispy snack.

HEALTHIER ALTERNATIVES.

For those mindful of fat content, you can experiment with part-skim milk to create a lower-fat version of mozzarella. This flexibility is one of the joys of making cheese at home.

PAIRING MOZZARELLA WITH OTHER HEALTHY FOODS.

Mozzarella pairs beautifully with a variety of healthy foods. Combine it with whole grains, fresh vegetables, or lean meats for balanced, nutritious meals.

THE THERAPEUTIC JOY OF CHEESE MAKING.

Beyond the nutritional benefits, the process of making mozzarella at home can be incredibly therapeutic and satisfying. It's a delightful way to connect with food and appreciate the art of cheese-making.

Embracing the Art of Homemade Mozzarella.

Homemade mozzarella is more than just cheese; it's a journey into the heart of traditional cooking, a celebration of natural ingredients, and a testament to the joy of creating something beautiful and nutritious with your own hands. In a world where processed foods are commonplace, taking the time to make something as simple and wholesome as mozzarella can be a deeply rewarding experience. Now, gather your ingredients, roll up your sleeves, and embark on the delightful adventure of making homemade mozzarella.

Detoxifying Natural Weight Loss Drinks.

The concept of detoxifying drinks for weight loss plays a melodious tune. These natural concoctions, often brimming with the goodness of herbs, fruits, and spices, are not just about shedding pounds; they are about nurturing the body, cleansing it from within, and restoring balance. We will search the world of detoxifying natural weight loss drinks, blending traditional wisdom with a sprinkle of modern understanding.

The Philosophy Behind Detoxification and Weight Loss.

Detoxification is a natural process where the body eliminates toxins. This process is crucial for optimal health and effective weight management. Detox drinks, therefore, are designed to support this natural process, aiding in digestion, boosting metabolism, and promoting overall health, which can subsequently aid in weight loss.

Key Ingredients in Detox Drinks.

- Lemon: A powerhouse of vitamin C, lemon aids in digestion and detoxification, helping to cleanse the liver and improve metabolism.

- Ginger: Known for its anti-inflammatory properties, ginger boosts digestion and warms the body, which can help in burning fat.

- Cucumber: High in water content and low in calories, cucumber is hydrating and helps to flush out toxins.

- Mint: Mint is not just a refreshing herb; it also promotes digestion and soothes the stomach.

81

- Apple Cider Vinegar: Rich in acetic acid, apple cider vinegar can boost metabolism and reduce water retention.

SIMPLE RECIPES FOR DETOX DRINKS.

- Lemon and Ginger Detox Water: Combine slices of lemon and ginger in a jar of water. Let it infuse overnight for a refreshing detox drink that stimulates digestion.

- Cucumber and Mint Water: Mix slices of cucumber and fresh mint leaves in water. This drink is perfect for staying hydrated and assisting in weight loss.

- Apple Cider Vinegar Tonic: Mix a tablespoon of apple cider vinegar with a glass of warm water. Add a touch of honey for sweetness and drink it in the morning to kickstart your metabolism.

THE ROLE OF DETOX DRINKS IN A HEALTHY LIFESTYLE.

Detox drinks are most effective when they are part of a balanced lifestyle that includes a nutritious diet and regular exercise. They are not magic potions but gentle aids that support the body's natural processes.

MINDFUL CONSUMPTION: QUALITY OVER QUANTITY.

When preparing and consuming detox drinks, it's essential to focus on quality. Use fresh, organic ingredients and consume these drinks as part of a balanced diet. It's not about the quantity but the quality and consistency.

Detox Drinks as Part of Your Daily Routine.

Integrating detox drinks into your daily routine can be a delightful experience. Start your day with a glass of lemon-ginger water or sip cucumber-mint water throughout the day for constant hydration and detoxification.

Understanding the Limitations and Precautions.

While detox drinks offer health benefits, they are not cure-alls. It's important to listen to your body and understand its limits. For instance, apple cider vinegar can be harsh on the teeth and stomach if consumed in excess.

Engaging with the Process: More Than Just Weight Loss.

The process of preparing and consuming these drinks should be seen as a ritual of self-care. It's an opportunity to slow down, engage with the ingredients, and savor the experience, reflecting a deeper appreciation for the body's needs.

A Symphony of Natural Wellness.

Detoxifying natural weight loss drinks are like a symphony of flavors and benefits, each ingredient playing its part in creating a harmonious blend that supports the body's natural detoxification processes and aids in weight management. These drinks are more than just weight loss aids; they are a celebration of nature's bounty and a testament to the gentle yet powerful ways we can support our health and well-being. As you sip on these refreshing, cleansing concoctions, remember that you're nurturing not just your body, but also your soul, tuning into the natural rhythms of health and wellness.

MINDFUL EATING: TRANSFORMING YOUR RELATIONSHIP WITH FOOD.

Mindful eating is like a dance of nourishment and awareness. This approach to food, far removed from the autopilot mode of rushed meals and distracted snacking, is a journey into the heart of true nourishment. We shall explore mindful eating, a practice that transforms our relationship with food, blending the rich traditions of mindful awareness with contemporary nutritional understanding.

THE ESSENCE OF MINDFUL EATING.

Mindful eating is about more than just slowing down or chewing your food thoroughly. It's an art that involves being fully present with each bite, savoring the flavors, and being attuned to the body's hunger and fullness cues. It's a practice rooted in mindfulness, a state of active, open attention to the present moment.

1. THE ORIGINS AND PHILOSOPHY OF MINDFUL EATING.

The concept of mindful eating has its roots in Buddhist teachings, which emphasize mindfulness as a path to enlightenment. In the context of eating, it's about experiencing food more intensely and consciously, thereby transforming the act of eating into a meditative practice.

2. THE BENEFITS OF MINDFUL EATING.

Mindful eating offers a cornucopia of benefits. It can help in managing weight, as it encourages you to eat slowly and recognize when you are full. It aids in digestion, as being mindful allows for better chewing and processing of food. It also enhances the joy of eating, as you fully engage with the textures and flavors of your meal.

THE PRACTICE OF MINDFUL EATING.

Engaging in mindful eating is an inviting and fulfilling practice. Here are some steps to get started:

- Sit Down and Eliminate Distractions: Dedicate a space for eating without the distractions of TV, phones, or computers.

- Engage All Your Senses: Before eating, take a moment to appreciate the colors, smells, textures, and even sounds of your food.

- Eat Slowly and Chew Thoroughly: Take your time with each bite, chewing slowly and thoroughly, allowing yourself to fully experience the flavors.

- Listen to Your Body: Pay attention to your hunger and fullness cues. Eat when you're hungry and stop when you're comfortably full.

INCORPORATING MINDFUL EATING INTO DAILY LIFE.

Transforming your relationship with food through mindful eating can be a gradual process. Start with one meal a day or even one snack. Use this time to practice eating with attention and intention.

MINDFUL EATING AND EMOTIONAL WELLNESS.

Mindful eating also means being aware of the emotional aspects of eating. It encourages you to explore the reasons behind your food choices and to be compassionate towards yourself, especially if you're eating in response to emotional needs.

CHALLENGES AND OVERCOMING THEM.

One of the challenges of mindful eating in today's fast-paced world is finding the time to eat mindfully. It is about quality, not quantity. Even a few mindful bites are better than a meal eaten in haste.

THE ROLE OF GRATITUDE IN MINDFUL EATING.

Incorporating a sense of gratitude into your meals can deepen the practice of mindful eating. Taking a moment to express gratitude for the food on your plate, and for the journey it took to get there, can enhance the eating experience.

A NOURISHING JOURNEY OF MINDFULNESS.

Mindful eating is more than a practice; it's a journey of rediscovering the joy and essence of nourishment. It encourages a harmonious relationship with food, where eating becomes an act of self-care and gratitude. Let each meal be an opportunity to engage with the present moment, to nourish not just the body, but also the soul, transforming the simple act of eating into a mindful, joyful experience.

Indoor Air Purifying Plants: Nature's Cleaners.

When we seek refuge and comfort, the air we breathe is often an overlooked aspect of our wellness. In the intricate ballet of indoor living, plants emerge not just as silent companions but as natural purifiers, gently cleansing the air we inhale. Let us look deeply into the enchanting world of indoor air purifying plants. These green wonders do more than beautify our spaces; they act as vigilant guardians of our health, subtly yet effectively enhancing the quality of our indoor environment.

The Science Behind Air Purifying Plants.

The journey of discovering indoor air purifying plants begins with understanding the science behind it. Studies by NASA and various environmental organizations have highlighted the ability of certain plants to filter out common volatile organic compounds (VOCs) such as benzene, formaldehyde, and trichloroethylene from the air. These toxins, often emitted by furniture, paints, and cleaning products, can contribute to what is known as 'sick building syndrome.'

Top Indoor Air Purifying Plants.

- Spider Plant (Chlorophytum comosum): A resilient and easy-to-care-for plant, the spider plant is known for its ability to remove formaldehyde and xylene from the air.

- Snake Plant (Sansevieria trifasciata): With its tall, upright leaves, the snake plant is not just an aesthetic addition but a potent air purifier, known for filtering out formaldehyde, trichloroethylene, benzene, and xylene. An added bonus is its ability to release oxygen at night, making it a perfect bedroom companion.

- Peace Lily (Spathiphyllum): This elegant plant is a powerhouse in removing airborne toxins, including ammonia, benzene, formaldehyde, and trichloroethylene. Its beautiful white blooms add a touch of serenity to any space.

- Aloe Vera: Besides its well-known skin-healing properties, aloe vera is effective in clearing formaldehyde and benzene from the air.

- Boston Fern (Nephrolepis exaltata): With its lush, feathery fronds, the Boston fern is a natural humidifier and a great remover of formaldehyde.

INTEGRATING PLANTS INTO YOUR HOME.

Incorporating air-purifying plants into your home is not just about placing a pot here and there. It's about creating a living ecosystem that contributes to the overall wellness of your indoor space.

- Strategic Placement: Place plants in areas where you spend most of your time, such as the living room, bedroom, and office space.

- Variety and Number: A variety of plants, distributed throughout your home, can maximize the air-purifying effect. NASA recommends having at least one plant per 100 square feet of home or office space.

- Caring for Your Plants: While these plants are generally low-maintenance, regular care, including watering, dusting the leaves, and occasional fertilizing, will keep them healthy and effective in air purification.

The Holistic Benefits of Indoor Plants.

Beyond purifying air, indoor plants offer holistic benefits. They bring a piece of nature into our homes, creating a calming and relaxing environment. This connection with nature can reduce stress, improve mood, and enhance cognitive function.

Mindfulness and Plants.

Caring for plants can be a mindful activity, a moment of connection with nature that reminds us of the cycles of growth and renewal. It's an opportunity to slow down, to nurture and be nurtured, much like the teachings of natural health advocates like Barbara O'Neill.

Embracing Nature's Gift for Healthier Living.

Indoor air purifying plants are nature's gift to our homes. They are silent, unassuming heroes that not only bring beauty and life into our indoor spaces but also protect and enhance our health. In this harmonious blend of greenery and wellness, we find a simple yet profound way of enhancing our daily lives, aligning with the natural wisdom that guides us towards healthier, more balanced living.

Natural Sleep Remedies for Restful Nights.

In a world bustling with the cacophony of modern life, the elusive embrace of sound sleep is often sought after. We shall examine natural sleep remedies, uncovering the secrets of nature's pharmacy to guide us into the arms of Morpheus. This journey is not just about finding sleep but about embracing a holistic approach to nighttime rejuvenation, blending time-honored traditions with modern insights into wellness.

Understanding the Importance of Sleep.

Before getting into the remedies, it's vital to understand why good sleep is crucial. Sleep is not just a passive state of rest but a dynamic process of restoration and healing. It's when the body repairs itself, the mind consolidates memories, and the spirit rejuvenates. Poor sleep can lead to a host of health issues, including weakened immunity, impaired cognitive function, and increased stress levels.

Herbal Allies for Sleep.

Nature's bounty offers a plethora of herbs that have been used for centuries to induce relaxation and sleep:

- Chamomile: Revered for its calming properties, chamomile tea is a bedtime favorite. Its gentle sedative effects come from the compound apigenin, which binds to certain receptors in the brain to reduce anxiety and initiate sleep.

- Lavender: The soothing aroma of lavender is more than just a pleasant scent. Inhaling lavender oil before bed can decrease stress levels and improve the quality of sleep, particularly in those with insomnia or anxiety.

- Valerian Root: Known as nature's valium, valerian root has been used for centuries to promote relaxation and sleep. It increases the levels of a neurotransmitter called GABA, which helps regulate nerve impulses in the brain and nervous system.

DIET AND SLEEP.

What we eat and drink can significantly impact our sleep quality:

- Warm Milk: A glass of warm milk before bed is not just a childhood ritual. Milk contains tryptophan, an amino acid that promotes the production of serotonin and melatonin, hormones that play a role in sleep.

- Almonds: Rich in magnesium, almonds can help improve sleep quality, especially for those who have insomnia. Magnesium's role in sleep involves regulating neurotransmitters that calm the body and mind.

- Bananas: Being a source of magnesium and potassium, bananas can relax overstressed muscles and provide tryptophan, aiding in a more restful night's sleep.

CREATING A SLEEP-INDUCING ENVIRONMENT.

The environment we sleep in profoundly affects our ability to fall and stay asleep:

- Reducing Electronic Distractions: Turn off electronic devices at least an hour before bedtime. The blue light emitted by screens can disrupt the production of melatonin, the hormone that regulates sleep cycles.

- Comfortable Bedding: Invest in comfortable mattresses and pillows. The physical comfort of your bed can significantly influence sleep quality.

- Aromatherapy: Using essential oils like lavender in a diffuser can create a calming ambiance conducive to sleep.

MINDFULNESS AND RELAXATION TECHNIQUES.

Mindfulness practices can greatly enhance sleep quality:

- Guided Meditation: Listening to guided meditations or sleep stories can help the mind unwind and drift into sleep.

- Deep Breathing Exercises: Techniques like the 4-7-8 breathing method can be a powerful tool to induce relaxation and sleep.

LIFESTYLE ADJUSTMENTS FOR BETTER SLEEP.

Incorporating certain lifestyle habits can significantly impact sleep patterns:

- Regular Exercise: Regular physical activity, especially in the morning or afternoon, can improve sleep quality and duration.

- Limiting Caffeine and Alcohol: Reducing intake of caffeine and alcohol, especially in the hours leading up to bedtime, can promote uninterrupted sleep.

EMBRACING NATURE'S NIGHTTIME SYMPHONY.

As we find these natural remedies for sleep, we not only get solutions for restful nights but also embrace a lifestyle that respects and aligns with our natural rhythms. Each remedy, be it a herb, a food, or a practice, plays its unique note in the symphony of sleep. By tuning into this natural rhythm, we learn not just to chase sleep but to invite it in, gently and naturally. So tonight, as you prepare for slumber, remember that sleep is not a mere pause but a rejuvenating journey, and nature has provided us with the most beautiful of maps to guide us through it.

Balancing Work, Health, and Life.

The quest for a harmonious balance between work, health, and life has become more than a mere aspiration; it is essential for our well-being. This adventure into balancing the various aspects of our lives is not just about dividing hours in a day but about weaving a pattern of life that resonates with health, happiness, and fulfillment. Let's blend the wisdom of old with the practicalities of our contemporary world, to master the art of balance in our lives.

Understanding the Need for Balance.

In our pursuit of career goals and personal ambitions, it's easy to overlook the importance of balance. Imbalance can lead to stress, burnout, and health issues, impacting our productivity and overall quality of life. Recognizing the signs of imbalance is the first step towards rectifying it.

1. The Role of Work in Our Lives.

Work is undoubtedly a significant part of our lives. It provides us with a sense of purpose, identity, and, of course, the means to support ourselves and our families. When work takes precedence over everything else, it can lead to an unhealthy lifestyle. Striking a balance between work and personal life is crucial for long-term happiness and health.

2. Health as a Foundation.

Health is the bedrock upon which the balance of work and life is built. Without good health, both work efficiency and life enjoyment can suffer. This includes physical health, mental well-being, and emotional stability.

Practical Strategies for Balancing Work and Health.

Finding balance doesn't require drastic changes; often, it's the small adjustments that make a big difference.

- Time Management: Prioritize your tasks and responsibilities. Learn to say no to unnecessary commitments and delegate tasks when possible.

- Work Boundaries: Set clear boundaries between work and personal time. This could mean turning off work emails after a certain hour or having a dedicated workspace that you can step away from.

- Regular Exercise: Incorporate physical activity into your daily routine. Exercise is not only good for physical health but also relieves stress and improves mental clarity.

- Mindful Eating: Pay attention to your diet. Nutritious food fuels both the body and mind, helping you to perform better in all aspects of life.

Embracing Mindfulness and Relaxation Techniques.

Incorporate mindfulness practices into your daily routine to reduce stress and improve focus. Techniques like meditation, deep breathing exercises, or yoga can be highly beneficial.

The Importance of Quality Sleep.

Never underestimate the power of good sleep. Quality sleep rejuvenates the body, enhances mood, and boosts productivity. Create a restful sleeping environment and establish a calming bedtime routine.

Cultivating a Supportive Social Network.

Having a supportive social circle; family, friends, or colleagues; is crucial. They can provide emotional support, practical help, and a different perspective on issues, which is invaluable for maintaining balance.

Finding Joy in Hobbies and Leisure Activities.

Engaging in hobbies and leisure activities that you enjoy can provide a much-needed break from work-related stress. It's essential to carve out time for activities that bring you joy, whether it's reading, gardening, painting, or anything else that fuels your passion.

Learning from Nature and Natural Rhythms.

Nature, in its wisdom, follows a rhythm; a balance of seasons, day and night, growth and rest. Observing and aligning with these natural rhythms can teach us valuable lessons about balance in our own lives.

Regular Health Check-Ups and Self-Care.

Regular health check-ups are vital for early detection and prevention of health issues. Equally important is self-care, which means taking time to care for your physical and mental health.

Weaving a Balanced Tapestry of Life.

Balancing work, health, and life is like weaving a tapestry with threads of different colors and textures. It requires patience, practice, and mindfulness. We learn that balance is not just about equal distribution of time but about harmonizing our activities with our body's needs, our mind's aspirations, and our soul's desires. As we blend these aspects seamlessly into our daily lives, we not only enhance our productivity and efficiency but also step into a space of greater peace, health, and fulfillment.

Soothing Herbal Teas for Relaxation and Health.

Herbal teas are gentle elixirs, soothing both body and soul. Enveloped in the warmth of a comforting cup, one finds more than just a beverage; one discovers a timeless ritual of relaxation and health. Let's embark on a delightful journey through the world of herbal teas.

The Healing Power of Herbal Teas.

Herbal teas, also known as tisanes, are not just aromatic infusions but are steeped in medicinal properties. Unlike traditional teas, which come from the Camellia sinensis plant, herbal teas are made from dried fruits, flowers, spices, or herbs. This means they are not only caffeine-free but also brimming with health-enhancing qualities.

1. Chamomile Tea: The Soother.

Chamomile, with its delicate white flowers, is renowned for its calming effects. A cup of chamomile tea can be a serene escape from the hustle of life, easing anxiety, promoting relaxation, and preparing the body for a restful sleep. Its gentle sedative effect is due to an antioxidant called apigenin, which binds to certain receptors in the brain.

2. Peppermint Tea: The Invigorator.

Peppermint tea, with its refreshing and cooling taste, is a wonderful digestive aid. It can relieve symptoms of bloating, cramping, and nausea, making it a comforting post-meal choice. The menthol in peppermint also makes it an ideal choice for clearing sinuses and relieving headaches.

3. Ginger Tea: The Healer.

Ginger tea, a zesty and warming brew, is famed for its anti-inflammatory properties. It aids digestion, soothes upset stomachs, and relieves nausea. Gingerol, the bioactive compound in ginger, also makes it effective in reducing muscle pain and soreness.

4. Lavender Tea: The Relaxant.

Lavender, with its mesmerizing aroma, is a balm for the nervous system. A cup of lavender tea can alleviate stress, reduce anxiety, and promote a peaceful night's sleep. Its calming properties also make it a great choice for soothing headaches and migraines.

5. Rooibos Tea: The Antioxidant Powerhouse.

Rooibos, a herb from South Africa, yields a naturally sweet and fruity tea. It's a treasure trove of antioxidants, which help in fighting free radicals and reducing the risk of chronic diseases. Rooibos is also known to promote healthy skin and hair.

CREATING THE PERFECT CUP OF HERBAL TEA.

Brewing herbal tea is an art that honors the essence of each herb:

- Quality Matters: Always start with high-quality, organic herbs. Freshness and purity of ingredients ensure maximum benefits and flavor.

- Water Temperature is Key: Unlike black or green teas, most herbal teas require boiling water to extract their full medicinal properties.

- Steeping Time: Steep your herbal tea for at least 5-10 minutes. This allows for a full extraction of the herbs' therapeutic properties.

INCORPORATING HERBAL TEAS INTO YOUR DAILY ROUTINE.

Herbal teas can be more than just occasional beverages; they can be woven into the fabric of your daily life:

- Morning Ritual: Start your day with a cup of ginger or peppermint tea to awaken your senses and stimulate digestion.

- Afternoon Pause: A cup of rooibos or fruit-infused herbal tea can be a refreshing afternoon treat.

- Evening Wind-Down: Make chamomile or lavender tea a part of your nightly routine to signal your body that it's time to unwind.

HERBAL TEAS AND EMOTIONAL WELLNESS.

Sipping on herbal tea can also be a moment of mindfulness and emotional healing. It allows a pause, a break from the digital world, offering a space to reflect, relax, and reconnect with oneself.

A JOURNEY TO WELLNESS IN EVERY CUP.

In every cup of herbal tea lies a journey into the heart of nature's healing wisdom. These soothing brews are not just about treating ailments but also about nurturing a state of balance and harmony within.

SEASONAL ALLERGIES: NATURAL REMEDIES THAT WORK.

As the seasons turn their pages, many of us find ourselves amidst the blossoming flora, only to be greeted by the less welcome arrival of seasonal allergies. The sneezes, the sniffles, the itchy eyes - they all seem like nature's taxing toll for enjoying its beauty. But fret not, for the same nature also holds the balm to soothe these seasonal woes. We shall identify some effective natural remedies for seasonal allergies, blending the wisdom of tradition with modern understanding.

UNDERSTANDING SEASONAL ALLERGIES.

Seasonal allergies, often known as hay fever, are the body's overreactive immune response to airborne substances like pollen. The body mistakes these harmless substances as threats, leading to an allergic reaction. Before diving into remedies, understanding this mechanism is crucial, as it helps in choosing the right natural treatments.

1. Neti Pot: A Traditional Nasal Irrigation Technique.

Originating from the Ayurvedic medical tradition, the Neti pot is a small teapot-like device used to rinse the nasal passages with a saltwater solution. This simple, yet effective practice clears the nasal passages of allergens and irritants, providing relief from congestion and reducing the severity of allergy symptoms.

2. Local Honey: Nature's Sweet Antidote.

Local honey, consumed regularly, can be a delightful remedy for seasonal allergies. The theory is that by ingesting honey produced by bees in your area, you can gradually become immune to the pollen that bees collect in your region. Start with small amounts daily before and during allergy season.

3. Quercetin: A Natural Antihistamine.

Quercetin, a flavonoid found in many fruits and vegetables, is known for its antihistamine properties. It stabilizes the release of histamines from certain immune cells, helping alleviate allergy symptoms. Foods rich in quercetin include apples, berries, grapes, onions, and black tea.

4. Butterbur: A Herbal Powerhouse.

Butterbur, a herb used historically for a variety of ailments, has shown promise in treating seasonal allergies. Studies suggest that it can be as effective as some antihistamine drugs without the drowsy side effects.

5. Stinging Nettle: An Herbal Antihistamine.

Stinging nettle, when taken in capsule or tea form, can naturally block the body's ability to produce histamine, offering relief from the typical allergy symptoms. It's a traditional remedy that's backed by some modern research.

6. Essential Oils: Aromatherapy for Allergy Relief.

Essential oils like peppermint, eucalyptus, and lavender can open up the airways, reduce inflammation, and create an environment less hospitable for allergens. Use them in a diffuser or apply them topically after diluting with a carrier oil.

7. Diet Changes: Reducing Inflammatory Foods.

A diet high in anti-inflammatory foods can help mitigate allergy symptoms. Incorporating omega-3 fatty acids, found in fish and flaxseed, and reducing consumption of inflammatory foods like processed sugars, can make a significant difference.

8. Acupuncture: An Ancient Approach.

Acupuncture, a key component of traditional Chinese medicine, involves inserting thin needles into specific points on the body. It's believed to help balance the body's energy pathways and could be beneficial for allergy sufferers.

9. Probiotics: Gut Health and Allergies.

Probiotics, found in fermented foods like yogurt, kefir, and sauerkraut, and also available as supplements, can strengthen the immune system. A healthy gut microbiome can play a crucial role in managing allergic reactions.

10. Stay Hydrated: Simple Yet Effective.

Sometimes, the simplest advice is the most effective. Staying well-hydrated keeps the mucous membranes moist, helping them trap and clear allergens more effectively.

EMBRACING NATURE'S REMEDIES.

As we journey through these natural pathways to alleviate seasonal allergies, it's a reminder of the profound wisdom inherent in nature and traditional practices. These remedies, offer us a way to harmonize with the seasons.

SUSTAINABLE GARDENING: GROWING HEALTH AT HOME.

In the heart of our homes lies a powerful source of health and wellness, often overlooked: our gardens. Sustainable gardening is not just about growing plants; it's about cultivating a healthier lifestyle and a deeper connection with nature. This practice, gives more than just fresh produce; it provides a sanctuary of well-being, right in our backyards.

THE ESSENCE OF SUSTAINABLE GARDENING.

Sustainable gardening involves practices that enrich the soil, conserve resources, and minimize negative impacts on the environment. It's about creating a garden that thrives naturally and harmoniously, mirroring the balance found in nature.

1. Start with Organic Soil.

Healthy gardening starts with healthy soil. Organic soil, rich in natural nutrients and microorganisms, is the foundation of a thriving garden. Composting kitchen scraps and yard waste can enrich your soil naturally, reducing the need for chemical fertilizers.

2. Choose Native Plants.

Native plants are adapted to the local climate and soil, requiring less water and maintenance. They also provide a natural habitat for local wildlife, promoting biodiversity in your garden.

3. Water Wisely.

Conserving water is a key aspect of sustainable gardening. Techniques like rainwater harvesting, drip irrigation, and mulching can significantly reduce water usage. Planting drought-tolerant species can also minimize the need for frequent watering.

4. Natural Pest Control.

Instead of chemical pesticides, embrace natural pest control methods. Companion planting, where certain plants are grown together for mutual benefit, can help deter pests. Encouraging beneficial insects like ladybugs and bees also aids in natural pest control and pollination.

5. Grow Your Food.

There's a unique joy in growing your own food. Vegetables and herbs grown in your garden are fresher, more nutritious, and free from harmful chemicals. Even a small balcony can be transformed into a mini vegetable garden.

6. Practice Crop Rotation.

Crop rotation, a practice of growing different types of crops in the same area in sequenced seasons, helps in maintaining soil health and reducing soil-borne diseases.

7. Embrace Seasonal Gardening.

Aligning your gardening practices with the seasons ensures that you work with nature, not against it. It allows you to grow a variety of produce and makes your garden more resilient.

8. Create a Wildlife-Friendly Garden.

A sustainable garden is a wildlife haven. By including features like bird feeders, birdbaths, and insect hotels, you can create a vibrant ecosystem that supports a variety of life.

9. Use Recycled Materials.

Sustainability is also about reducing waste. Using recycled materials for planters, borders, and garden art not only adds character to your garden but also helps the environment.

10. Educate and Share.

Sharing your sustainable gardening journey with others can inspire more people to adopt eco-friendly practices. Community gardens, workshops, and social media are great platforms to spread this green wisdom.

A GARDEN OF HEALTH AND HARMONY.

Sustainable gardening is more than just a hobby; it's a lifestyle that nurtures both personal and environmental well-being. As we tend to our gardens, we are reminded of the simplicity and richness of life, the joy of connecting with the earth, and the profound satisfaction of growing our health. In every seed planted and every plant nurtured, lies the potential for a healthier, more sustainable world.

DAILY GRATITUDE: ENHANCING HEALTH AND HAPPINESS.

In the hustle and bustle of modern life, we often overlook the simple yet profound practice of gratitude. This humble act, deeply rooted in various cultural and spiritual traditions holds the key to transforming our health and happiness.

THE ESSENCE OF GRATITUDE.

Gratitude goes beyond saying 'thank you.' It's an emotional state, a way of perceiving and experiencing life. It incorporates recognizing the value in the simple things and acknowledging the abundance already present in our lives.

1. Gratitude and Physical Health.

Studies have shown that gratitude can have a tangible effect on physical health. People who practice gratitude regularly often experience fewer aches and pains and report feeling healthier than others. Gratitude also contributes to heart health by reducing blood pressure and improving cardiac functioning.

2. Mental Health Benefits.

Gratitude is a powerful tool for mental health. It can reduce a multitude of toxic emotions, ranging from envy and resentment to frustration and regret. Practicing gratitude increases happiness and reduces depression. It's a natural antidepressant that triggers positive feedback loops in our brains.

3. Gratitude for Better Sleep.

Writing in a gratitude journal before bed can help improve sleep quality. Spending just 15 minutes jotting down a few grateful sentiments before bed may help you sleep better and longer. This practice helps in winding down and reflecting on the positives of the day.

4. Improved Self-Esteem.

A 2014 study published in the Journal of Applied Sport Psychology found that gratitude increased athletes' self-esteem, an essential component for optimal performance. Instead of becoming resentful towards people who have more, gratitude helps people appreciate other people's accomplishments.

5. Enhances Empathy and Reduces Aggression.

Gratitude can help us become more empathetic and less aggressive. Grateful people are more likely to behave in a prosocial manner, even when others behave less kind. They experience more sensitivity and empathy towards other people and a decreased desire to seek revenge.

6. Building Resilience.

Practicing gratitude helps in building psychological resilience, making us more resilient to traumatic events. It's not about ignoring the hardships but about finding a silver lining, which is crucial in the face of adversity.

7. Strengthening Relationships.

Showing appreciation can help you win new friends, according to a 2014 study published in Emotion. Thanking a new acquaintance makes them more likely to seek an ongoing relationship. Gratitude also strengthens existing relationships.

8. Gratitude in the Workplace.

A workplace that practices gratitude tends to have a more cooperative and collaborative work environment. Recognizing the good work of colleagues and expressing thanks can contribute to a more positive work culture.

9. Simple Ways to Practice Gratitude.

Start with small steps like keeping a gratitude journal, saying thank you more often, meditating, and focusing on positive thoughts. Even in challenging times, try to find one thing to be grateful for each day.

10. Gratitude and Spirituality.

For many, gratitude is deeply connected to their spiritual beliefs. It's about acknowledging the goodness in their lives and understanding that the source of this goodness lies at least partially outside themselves.

EMBRACING GRATITUDE IN EVERYDAY LIFE.

Incorporating gratitude into our daily lives isn't just a nicety; it's a necessity for a fulfilling life. It's about changing our perspective, focusing on abundance rather than lack, and recognizing the wealth of blessings we often overlook. Let's not wait for the perfect moment to be grateful; let's make every moment perfect with our gratitude.

JOINT PAIN: NATURAL RELIEF STRATEGIES.

Joint pain, a common ailment that plagues many, often leads us down a path of conventional medications and treatments. Yet, in the teachings of natural health advocates like Barbara O'Neill, we find a treasure trove of alternative, natural strategies for alleviating joint discomfort.

UNDERSTANDING JOINT PAIN.

It is pivotal to understand what causes joint pain. It can arise from a variety of factors, including arthritis, age-related wear and tear, overuse, or injury. The pain can range from mildly irritating to debilitating, affecting one's quality of life.

1. The Power of Anti-Inflammatory Foods.

One of the most effective ways to combat joint pain naturally is through diet. Foods rich in anti-inflammatory properties can significantly reduce joint inflammation. Turmeric, with its active compound curcumin, ginger, omega-3 rich foods like salmon and flaxseeds, and antioxidants found in berries, can all contribute to reducing inflammation.

2. Herbal Remedies.

Herbs have been used for centuries to treat various ailments, including joint pain. Herbs like devil's claw, boswellia, and stinging nettle have shown promise in reducing joint pain and inflammation.

3. The Magic of Movement.

While it may seem counterintuitive, regular gentle exercise can help alleviate joint pain. Activities like walking, swimming, or yoga can strengthen the muscles around the joints, improve flexibility, and reduce pain.

4. The Role of Weight Management.

Excess weight can put additional stress on weight-bearing joints like the hips and knees. Losing weight, even a small amount, can significantly reduce joint pain and prevent further joint damage.

5. Heat and Cold Therapy.

Applying heat or cold to the affected joints can provide immediate pain relief. Heat therapy helps in relaxing muscles and increasing blood flow, while cold therapy can reduce inflammation and numb the pain.

6. Massage Therapy.

Massage can be a therapeutic option for joint pain relief. It can help in increasing blood circulation, reducing stiffness, and improving range of motion.

7. Acupuncture.

Acupuncture, a staple in traditional Chinese medicine, can also offer relief from joint pain. It involves inserting thin needles into specific points on the body, which can help in releasing endorphins and triggering anti-inflammatory responses.

8. Essential Oils.

Essential oils like lavender, eucalyptus, and peppermint have analgesic and anti-inflammatory properties. Used in aromatherapy or applied topically, they can provide relief from joint discomfort.

9. Hydrotherapy.

Water exercises or even a warm bath can be beneficial for joint pain. The buoyancy of water reduces stress on the joints, and the warmth can soothe the pain.

10. Mind-Body Techniques.

Practices like meditation, deep breathing, and mindfulness can help in managing the pain by reducing stress and improving one's coping mechanisms.

11. Supplements.

Certain supplements can be beneficial in managing joint pain. Glucosamine and chondroitin, omega-3 fatty acids, and green tea extract are some supplements known for their joint health benefits.

12. Topical Treatments.

Applying creams or gels containing capsaicin or menthol directly to the affected joints can provide temporary relief by blocking pain signals.

13. Sleep and Joint Health.

Adequate sleep is crucial for overall health and can also impact joint pain. Poor sleep can exacerbate pain, while good sleep habits can improve pain management.

A Holistic Approach to Joint Pain.

Managing joint pain naturally includes focusing on diet, lifestyle changes, and natural remedies. These methods do not only relieve pain but also improve overall health and well-being. It's about listening to our bodies and treating them with the care and respect they deserve. Each individual's response to these remedies can vary, so it's necessary to find what works best for you and consult with healthcare professionals when necessary.

Heart-Healthy Eating for a Vibrant Life.

Our hearts, those tirelessly working engines, deserve the best fuel for a vibrant, healthy life. Here, we search how simple, heart-healthy dietary changes can be profoundly rewarding.

Understanding the Heart's Needs.

Our heart, a marvel of nature, thrives on specific nutrients. Just like a garden that requires the right balance of sun, water, and nutrients, our heart needs a balanced diet rich in certain foods to function optimally. This includes whole grains, healthy fats, and a bounty of fruits and vegetables.

1. The Whole Grain Goodness.

Incorporating whole grains into our diet is like laying a strong foundation. Whole grains like oats, barley, and brown rice are rich in fiber, which helps in lowering bad cholesterol, a nemesis of heart health. A bowl of oatmeal or whole-grain bread can be both comforting and heart-protective.

2. Fruits and Vegetables: Nature's Palette.

A diet rich in fruits and vegetables is akin to painting our plate with nature's colors. These food items are not only visually pleasing but are also packed with vitamins, minerals, and antioxidants that support heart health. The mantra here is variety; from leafy greens to bright berries, each brings its unique heart benefits.

3. The Magic of Healthy Fats.

Healthy fats, particularly omega-3 fatty acids found in fish like salmon and mackerel, are like lubricants for the heart. They aid in reducing inflammation and lowering the risk of heart rhythm disorders. Plant-based sources like flaxseeds and walnuts are also beneficial.

4. The Spice of Life.

Spices not only add flavor but can also boost heart health. Turmeric, with its curcumin content, and ginger, with its anti-inflammatory properties, are like natural supplements for the heart.

5. Hydration: The Elixir of Life.

Water, the most basic yet essential element, plays a critical role in maintaining heart health. Adequate hydration helps in efficient circulation and keeping blood pressure in check.

6. Reducing Salt: A Small Step with Big Impact.

Cutting down on salt can have a significant impact on heart health. High salt intake is linked to high blood pressure, a risk factor for heart disease. Using herbs and spices for flavoring can be a delightful alternative.

7. Limiting Processed Foods: Back to Basics.

Processed foods are often high in unhealthy fats, salt, and sugar - enemies of the heart. Embracing whole, unprocessed foods is not only heart-friendly but also reconnects us with the joys of basic, natural eating.

8. The Role of Fermented Foods.

Fermented foods like yogurt and kefir are beneficial for heart health due to their probiotic content. They help in maintaining a healthy gut microbiome, which is surprisingly linked to heart health.

9. The Power of Portion Control.

Eating in moderation is as important as choosing the right foods. Portion control helps in maintaining a healthy weight, crucial for heart health.

10. The Joy of Cooking at Home.

Cooking at home allows for control over ingredients and preparation methods, making it easier to adhere to a heart-healthy diet. It's also a delightful way to nurture oneself and loved ones.

11. Mindful Eating: A Heartful Approach.

Mindful eating, a concept often highlighted by Barbara O'Neill, involves being present and attentive to our food choices and eating habits. It's about enjoying each bite and recognizing the nourishing qualities of food.

12. Embracing Variety.

A heart-healthy diet doesn't have to be monotonous. Exploring different cuisines and ingredients can make eating for heart health an exciting culinary adventure.

A JOURNEY TO HEART HEALTH.

Adopting a heart-healthy diet is not just about avoiding certain foods; it's a journey towards a more vibrant, healthful life. Each meal is an opportunity to nourish and cherish our hearts. This means making choices that resonate with our body's natural rhythms and needs, all while enjoying the bountiful pleasures of natural, wholesome foods.

FOODS THAT NATURALLY COMBAT STRESS.

In a world where stress seems as common as the air we breathe, it's a breath of fresh air to learn that nature has provided us with foods that can help manage and reduce stress. I would often echo Barbara O'Neill's teachings on using nature's bounty for holistic well-being. Let's set out on this delightful journey to discover how certain foods can be our allies in the battle against stress.

UNDERSTANDING STRESS AND ITS IMPACT.

Stress, that unwelcome yet familiar visitor, can wreak havoc on our physical and mental well-being. It's like a storm that disrupts the calm seas of our lives. But just as storms can be weathered, so can stress, with the right nutritional choices.

1. The Soothing Power of Leafy Greens.

Leafy greens such as spinach and kale are like a soothing balm for the stressed mind. Rich in folate, they help produce mood-regulating neurotransmitters like serotonin and dopamine. It's like turning on a light in a dark room.

2. The Magic of Omega-3 Fatty Acids.

Foods like salmon, flaxseeds, and walnuts are not just a treat for the taste buds but also for the brain. Omega-3 fatty acids in these foods are known to reduce stress hormones and inflammation, much like a gentle wave smoothing over ripples in the sand.

3. The Comfort of Whole Grains.

Whole grains, in their unrefined glory, are rich in fiber, which helps regulate blood sugar levels. Steady blood sugar levels mean a steady mood, making whole grains a comforting, stress-reducing choice.

4. The Antioxidant Richness of Berries.

Berries, with their vibrant colors and sweet taste, are not just a feast for the eyes but also a potent source of antioxidants. These nutrients combat oxidative stress, offering a shield against the wear and tear of stress on the body.

5. The Calming Effect of Herbal Teas.

A cup of herbal tea, be it chamomile, peppermint, or lavender, is like a warm, comforting hug. These teas have natural calming properties that can help soothe a stressed mind and body.

6. The Soothing Nature of Dark Chocolate.

Dark chocolate, rich in antioxidants and magnesium, can be a delightful way to reduce stress. It's like a sweet whisper telling you that everything will be alright.

7. The Power of Probiotics.

Fermented foods like yogurt, kefir, and sauerkraut are not just for the gut but also for the mind. Probiotics in these foods help improve gut health, which is closely linked to mental health.

8. The Strength of Seeds.

Seeds like pumpkin, sunflower, and chia are tiny powerhouses of magnesium and tryptophan, which help in the production of serotonin, a feel-good neurotransmitter. They are like little sparks of joy in the fight against stress.

9. The Hydration Factor.

Sometimes, simply staying hydrated can help manage stress. Water, herbal teas, and natural fruit juices keep the body well-hydrated, ensuring all systems function optimally, thereby reducing the physical effects of stress.

10. The Spice of Life.

Spices such as turmeric and ginger not only add flavor to our food but also have anti-inflammatory and antioxidant properties. Incorporating these spices into our diet can be a simple yet effective way to combat stress.

11. The Balancing Act of Complex Carbohydrates.

Foods like sweet potatoes and quinoa, rich in complex carbohydrates, help produce serotonin, offering a mood boost. It's like adding a steady rhythm to the chaotic melody of life.

NOURISHING THE BODY AND MIND.

Incorporating these stress-busting foods into our daily diet is a form of self-care and self-love. As I would say, each meal is an opportunity to nourish not just our bodies but also our souls. Eating these foods mindfully, savoring each bite, can transform our relationship with food from mere sustenance to a joyful, stress-reducing experience.

Meditation for Everyday Calm.

Meditation is a gentle yet profound melody that soothes the soul and calms the mind. I often emphasize the transformative power of meditation in nurturing overall well-being. Let's see how integrating meditation into our daily routine can be a gateway to tranquility and balance.

Understanding Meditation and Its Roots.

Meditation, a practice as ancient as time itself, is the art of focusing one's mind to achieve a mentally clear and emotionally calm state. It's akin to finding a quiet corner in a bustling market; a place of peace amid chaos.

The Science Behind Meditation.

Modern research echoes what ancient wisdom has always known: meditation has profound effects on the mind and body. It's like a key that unlocks the door to reduced stress, enhanced focus, and improved emotional well-being.

Simple Steps to Begin Your Meditation Journey.

- Finding a Quiet Space: Just as a seed needs fertile soil to grow, meditation requires a quiet space. It need not be elaborate; a small corner in your home where you can sit undisturbed is perfect.

- Setting a Time: Consistency is key. Whether it's the first rays of the morning sun or the quiet of the evening, choose a time that suits you and stick to it.

- Comfortable Positioning: Sit comfortably, whether on a chair or cross-legged on the floor, with your back straight yet relaxed. It's like settling into a cozy armchair with your favorite book.

- Focusing on the Breath: Your breath is a powerful tool. Pay attention to the rhythm of your breathing; inhale and exhale naturally. It's like watching the gentle ebb and flow of ocean waves.

- Letting Go of Thoughts: As thoughts come, let them float away like leaves on a stream. The goal is not to empty the mind but to observe without attachment.

- Starting with Short Sessions: Begin with 5-10 minutes and gradually increase. It's like savoring a fine tea; you start with small sips and gradually immerse yourself in its flavors.

THE MANY FORMS OF MEDITATION.

- Mindfulness Meditation: This involves being fully present and aware of your surroundings. It's like walking in a garden and noticing every flower and leaf.

- Guided Meditation: Here, you visualize a relaxing place or scenario with the guidance of a teacher or an app. It's akin to following a gentle voice through a serene forest.

- Mantra Meditation: In this style, you silently repeat a calming word or phrase to prevent distracting thoughts. It's like a soft, repetitive melody that brings you back to calmness.

- Yoga and Movement Meditation: This combines meditation with yoga or other forms of gentle movement, enhancing the connection between mind and body.

Integrating Meditation into Daily Life.

- Morning Ritual: Start your day with meditation to set a peaceful tone for what lies ahead.

- Mindful Moments: Practice mindfulness during everyday activities like eating, walking, or even while doing chores.

- Evening Unwind: A short meditation session in the evening can help release the day's stress and prepare you for restful sleep.

Overcoming Challenges in Meditation.

It's common to face hurdles like restlessness, drowsiness, or a wandering mind. The key is to approach meditation with patience and kindness towards oneself. It's not about perfection but progression.

A Journey to Inner Peace.

Meditation is a journey that takes you deeper into inner peace and serenity. It centers on finding moments of calm in a world that often moves too fast. Embracing meditation is not just about reducing stress; it's about enriching your life with clarity, joy, and a profound sense of being connected to the world around you. Let each breath be a step towards a calmer you.

Immunity-Boosting Strategies from Nature.

Turning to nature for immunity-boosting strategies seems like returning to our roots. We will examine how nature's bounty can be our ally in building a robust immune system.

Understanding Immunity and Its Importance.

Immunity is the body's shield against diseases. It's a complex system that acts like a vigilant guardian, constantly protecting us from harmful pathogens. Strengthening it is akin to fortifying the walls of a castle.

Nature's Pharmacy: Immunity-Boosting Heroes.

- Echinacea: Known for its vibrant purple flowers, Echinacea has been used traditionally to combat colds and flu. It's like nature's warrior, ready to defend at the first sign of an invasion.

- Ginger: With its zesty flavor, ginger not only adds zest to dishes but also boosts immunity. Its warming property is like a cozy blanket on a chilly day, offering comfort and protection.

- Garlic: This humble kitchen staple is a powerhouse for enhancing immune function. Think of garlic as an old, wise sage with potent secrets.

- Turmeric: With its golden hue, turmeric is not just for adding color to curries. Its active compound, curcumin, is like a magic wand, waving off inflammation and boosting immunity.

- Green Tea: Loaded with antioxidants, green tea is like a gentle brook, cleansing and refreshing the body.

INCORPORATING NATURE'S REMEDIES INTO DAILY LIFE.

- Herbal Teas: Create a daily ritual of sipping herbal teas. It's like a daily meeting with nature, discussing how to keep you healthy.

- Cooking with Spices: Add ginger, garlic, and turmeric to your meals. It's like inviting a team of health guardians to your dining table.

- Supplements: In times when fresh herbs are not available, supplements can be a convenient alternative. It's like having a backup plan for your immune system.

LIFESTYLE PRACTICES TO COMPLEMENT NATURAL REMEDIES.

- Adequate Sleep: Ensure you get enough sleep. Think of it as recharging your body's batteries.

- Stress Management: Practice yoga, meditation, or any activity that reduces stress. It's like smoothing out the wrinkles of worry from your body.

- Regular Exercise: Keep your body active. It's like taking your immune system for a joyful dance.

THE ROLE OF DIET IN BOOSTING IMMUNITY.

- Fruits and Vegetables: Consume a rainbow of fruits and vegetables. Each color brings its unique set of nutrients, like a palette of health.

- Probiotics and Prebiotics: Include foods rich in probiotics and prebiotics for gut health, which is closely linked to immunity.

- Balanced Nutrition: Ensure a well-balanced diet to provide your body with all the essential nutrients. It's like building a strong foundation for your health castle.

OVERCOMING OBSTACLES IN NATURAL IMMUNITY BUILDING.

The path to natural immunity enhancement is not always straightforward. One may face challenges like allergies to certain herbs or the availability of ingredients. The key is to listen to your body and adjust according to what works best for you in the vast garden of natural remedies.

A JOURNEY TOWARDS HEALTHIER LIVING.

Embracing nature's remedies for boosting immunity is means creating a harmonious relationship between our bodies and the natural world. The secrets to a strong immune system lie in the simplicity of nature and our willingness to embrace it. So, let us take this knowledge and embark on a journey of health and vitality, one natural remedy at a time.

Healthy Aging: Nature's Secrets for Longevity

Aging gracefully is a journey best accompanied by nature's wisdom, aging isn't a process to fight against but an experience to embrace with the help of nature's secrets. This section explains natural strategies for promoting healthy aging and longevity.

Understanding Aging and Its Natural Process.

Aging is as natural as the changing seasons. It's a process that brings its own beauty and challenges. Embracing it requires understanding the role of genetics, lifestyle, and the environment.

Nature's Bounty: Allies for Healthy Aging.

- Antioxidant-Rich Foods: Fruits and vegetables like blueberries, spinach, and nuts are packed with antioxidants. They're like nature's little cleaners, sweeping away harmful free radicals.

- Omega-3 Fatty Acids: Found in fish, flaxseeds, and walnuts, omega-3s are like lubricants for the body, ensuring everything runs smoothly, especially heart health.

- Herbs and Spices: Turmeric, ginger, and garlic aren't just flavor enhancers. They're like nature's medicine, reducing inflammation and supporting overall health.

- Water: Hydration is key at every age. Drinking water is like giving your body a fresh, clear stream to rejuvenate itself.

LIFESTYLE PRACTICES TO COMPLEMENT NATURE'S OFFERINGS.

- Regular Physical Activity: Exercise isn't just about staying fit. It's like a tonic for the mind, body, and soul, keeping everything in harmony.

- Mindfulness and Meditation: Practices like yoga and meditation are more than relaxation techniques. They're paths to inner peace, aligning mind, body, and spirit.

- Adequate Sleep: Restorative sleep is like pressing the reset button, giving your body time to heal and rejuvenate.

INCORPORATING NATURAL REMEDIES INTO DAILY LIFE.

- Balanced Diet: Eating a diet rich in fruits, vegetables, lean proteins, and whole grains is like building a strong fort, offering protection against age-related ailments.

- Healthy Fats: Incorporating healthy fats from sources like avocados and olive oil is like adding a layer of protection for your heart and brain.

- Reducing Sugar and Processed Foods: Limiting these is like reducing noise pollution, allowing your body to function more peacefully and efficiently.

Overcoming Challenges in Embracing Natural Aging.

Adapting to a natural lifestyle for aging can have its hurdles, such as dietary restrictions or accessibility to certain foods. The key is flexibility and finding what works for your unique body.

Embracing Aging with Nature's Help.

Embracing aging with the help of nature is about creating a harmonious relationship with our own bodies and the world around us. The key to longevity lies not in fighting aging but in embracing it with grace, using the tools provided by nature. It's about nurturing our bodies with natural foods, engaging in physical and mental wellness practices, and appreciating the beauty of aging.

Natural Detox: Gentle Ways to Rejuvenate.

In our bustling lives, we often forget the wisdom of nature in maintaining our health and vitality. Gentle detoxification using natural methods can be a powerful tool to rejuvenate our bodies and minds.

Understanding the Need for Natural Detox.

Our bodies are naturally equipped to detoxify, but in today's world, with its pollution and processed foods, this system can be overwhelmed. A gentle, natural detox aids our body's innate ability to cleanse itself.

The Foundations of Gentle Detoxification.

- Hydration with a Twist: Water is the essence of life, and for a detox, infusing it with lemon, cucumber, or herbs can enhance its cleansing properties.

- The Power of Green: Incorporating leafy greens like spinach and kale into our diet is akin to giving our body a natural cleanse with every bite.

- Fiber-Rich Foods: Whole grains, fruits, and vegetables act like gentle scrubbers in our digestive tract, helping to eliminate toxins.

Herbal Allies in Detoxification.

Herbs like milk thistle, dandelion root, and nettle have been used for centuries to support liver and kidney function, the cornerstones of detoxification.

Mindful Eating for Detox.

Mindful eating is not just about what we eat but how we eat. Slowing down and chewing thoroughly aids digestion and absorption, key components of detoxification.

Gentle Movement for Effective Detox.

Exercise need not be strenuous. Gentle practices like yoga and walking stimulate blood circulation and lymphatic drainage, supporting the body's natural detox processes.

The Role of Restful Sleep.

Sleep is when our body repairs and detoxifies. Ensuring quality sleep is ensuring a natural nightly detox.

Embracing Traditional Wisdom.

Detoxification is not a new concept. Traditional practices like dry skin brushing, oil pulling, and sauna use are time-honored methods that still hold relevance today.

Detox Through Hydration.

Starting the day with warm water and lemon is like a gentle wake-up call for the digestive system, preparing it for the day's detoxification tasks.

Natural Detox with Foods and Herbs.

Incorporating detoxifying foods like garlic, ginger, and cruciferous vegetables into our diet can be a delicious way to cleanse our system.

The Power of Simplicity.

In detoxification, sometimes less is more. Simple meals, simple ingredients, and a simple lifestyle can sometimes be the most effective detox strategy.

Mindful Lifestyle Choices.

Detoxification is not just about food. Reducing exposure to toxins in our environment, from cleaning products to personal care items, can significantly impact our body's detoxification efforts.

A Holistic Approach to Detox.

Detox is not just a physical process; it's an emotional and spiritual one too. Practices like meditation and gratitude can help cleanse our minds and spirits.

A Journey to Rejuvenation.

Detoxification is about rejuvenating and nurturing our bodies and minds through nature's wisdom and returning to the basics of hydration, nutrition, movement, and rest. It's about living in a way that supports our body's natural processes and practising the powerful methods that nature offers to rejuvenate and restore balance.

YOGA FOR EVERY BODY: FLEXIBILITY AND STRENGTH.

Yoga, a practice as ancient as time itself, is not just as a form of exercise but as a holistic approach to achieving balance and harmony within ourselves. Let us unravel the beauty of yoga and discover how it can bring flexibility and strength to everybody, regardless of age or fitness level.

THE ESSENCE OF YOGA.

Yoga, at its core, is about unity - the harmonious connection of mind, body, and spirit. It's a practice that goes beyond physical postures; it's a way of living. Through yoga, we learn to listen to our bodies, respect our limits, and gently push boundaries, leading to growth and transformation.

YOGA FOR FLEXIBILITY.

One of the most visible benefits of yoga is improved flexibility. Many people shy away from yoga, thinking they're not flexible enough, but yoga is not about touching your toes; it's about what you learn on the way down. Gentle stretches and poses gradually increase your range of motion, reducing stiffness and pain.

YOGA FOR STRENGTH.

Yoga is also about building strength - both physical and mental. Each pose requires a balance of effort and ease, engaging muscles and building core strength. This physical strength is mirrored in our mental resilience, as yoga teaches us to persevere through challenges, both on and off the mat.

Adapting Yoga for Every Body.

Yoga is inclusive. Whether you're a seasoned practitioner or a beginner, there are poses and modifications for every level. Props like blocks and straps can help make poses accessible. It's about finding what works for your body.

The Breath Connection.

In yoga, breath is everything. It's the bridge between body and mind. Learning to breathe deeply and consciously brings a sense of calm and focus, essential for both flexibility and strength.

Yoga and Mindfulness.

Yoga is a practice of mindfulness. Each pose is an opportunity to tune into the present moment. This awareness transcends the mat, helping us navigate life with a sense of peace and presence.

The Role of Yoga in Holistic Health.

Barbara O'Neill, a proponent of holistic health, often emphasizes the importance of integrating body and mind practices for overall well-being. Yoga perfectly aligns with this philosophy, offering a way to balance our physical health with our mental and emotional needs.

Starting Your Yoga Journey.

Beginning a yoga practice can be as simple as rolling out a mat in your living room. Many online resources and local classes cater to beginners. The key is to start slow and be consistent.

Yoga's Healing Power.

The therapeutic aspects of yoga are well-documented. From reducing stress to alleviating chronic conditions, yoga has the power to heal and rejuvenate.

Yoga as a Lifestyle.

Beyond physical practice, yoga is a way of life. It teaches kindness, patience, and gratitude - principles that enhance our daily lives and interactions with others.

A Path to Harmony.

Yoga is a path that leads to improved flexibility, increased strength, and a deeper connection with ourselves. Health is not just the absence of disease; it's a state of complete physical, mental, and social well-being. Yoga offers a holistic approach to achieving this state, making it a valuable practice for everyone seeking a vibrant and balanced life.

Mental Clarity: Natural Techniques for Focus.

The quest for mental clarity is akin to finding a serene oasis in a desert. As a proponent of natural health, I've discovered that achieving focus and clarity doesn't require modern gimmicks; instead, it's about reconnecting with the timeless wisdom of nature. We are going to identify natural techniques to enhance focus and clear the mind.

The Power of Nature's Silence.

Firstly, embracing the quietude of nature is a potent tool. In our technology-driven lives, we're bombarded with constant noise and distractions. Stepping into the calm of a forest or sitting by a serene lake can be transformative. It's in these moments of stillness that our minds can declutter and refocus.

Herbal Allies for Focus.

Herbs have long been our allies in health and well-being. Certain herbs like Ginkgo Biloba, known for enhancing cerebral blood flow, and Rosemary, with its memory-boosting properties, can be invaluable. A simple herbal tea or aromatherapy session using these plants can work wonders for mental clarity.

Breathing Techniques for Concentration.

Breath, the essence of life, is a powerful tool for achieving mental clarity. Practices such as deep belly breathing or the balanced 'Pranayama' techniques from yoga help oxygenate the brain and sharpen focus. These breathing exercises, often overlooked, are simple yet effective ways to clear mental fog.

THE ART OF MINDFULNESS.

Mindfulness, a practice that Barbara O'Neill often highlights for overall well-being, is also crucial for mental clarity. Being fully present in the moment, whether it's while eating, walking, or even during mundane tasks, helps train the brain to focus. Mindfulness is not just a practice but a way of living, bringing clarity to every moment of our lives.

NOURISHING THE BRAIN WITH THE RIGHT FOODS.

Diet plays a significant role in cognitive function. Foods rich in Omega-3 fatty acids like walnuts and flaxseeds, antioxidants found in berries, and the brain-boosting compounds in dark chocolate, can enhance focus and clarity. A balanced diet, full of whole foods, is not just for physical health, but mental as well.

PHYSICAL EXERCISE FOR MENTAL SHARPNESS.

Physical activity is as crucial for the mind as it is for the body. Regular exercise, especially aerobic activities like walking or swimming, boosts blood flow to the brain, which in turn improves cognitive functions and concentration.

RESTORATIVE SLEEP FOR A CLEAR MIND.

Never underestimate the power of good sleep. Sleep is the time when our brain processes information, consolidates memories, and rejuvenates. Ensuring a restful sleep routine, possibly enhanced with calming herbs like lavender, is essential for mental clarity.

Hydration: The Simplest Key to Focus.

Water is life, and this isn't just a saying. Keeping hydrated is one of the simplest yet most effective ways to maintain mental sharpness. Dehydration can lead to confusion and reduced cognitive function, so drinking ample water throughout the day is crucial.

Digital Detox for a Clearer Mind.

In our digital age, one of the best things we can do for our minds is occasionally disconnecting. A digital detox, even if just for a few hours, can reduce stress and improve concentration.

Embracing Nature's Wisdom.

Achieving mental clarity and focus is less about complex techniques and more about embracing the simple, natural wisdom that surrounds us. Sometimes, the answers lie in going back to the basics. By incorporating these natural strategies into our daily lives, we can enhance our mental clarity, focus, and overall well-being.

DIY Natural Beauty: Makeup and Skin Care.

In the embrace of nature, we find not only solace but also a treasure trove of beauty secrets. The art of DIY natural beauty, a blend of old wisdom and new understanding, offers us a way to care for our skin and enhance our beauty with the purest of ingredients. Let's look into the world of homemade makeup and skincare, where every ingredient has a purpose and every creation is a step towards natural wellness.

The Essence of Natural Ingredients.

In our journey towards natural beauty, the first step is understanding the power of simple, pure ingredients. Herbs, essential oils, and everyday kitchen staples hold the key to effective and gentle beauty solutions. It's about rekindling a connection with the earth, much like Barbara O'Neil advocates, to nurture our skin and body.

Creating Your Own Skincare Elixirs.

Why not start with homemade facial cleansers? For instance, a combination of honey, known for its antibacterial properties, and oatmeal, an excellent natural exfoliant, can create a gentle yet effective cleanser suitable for all skin types. These natural ingredients not only cleanse but also nourish the skin, leaving it radiant and soft.

The Magic of Herbal Toners.

Toners are an essential step in any skincare routine, and creating them at home is both simple and gratifying. A rosewater and witch hazel toner, for instance, can soothe and balance the skin, providing a refreshing burst of natural fragrance. These herbal concoctions are not just skincare products but a daily ritual of self-care.

Nourishing Homemade Masks.

Facial masks are a wonderful way to deep cleanse and rejuvenate the skin. A simple avocado and yogurt mask can hydrate and exfoliate, leaving the skin feeling refreshed and alive. These natural masks, enriched with vitamins and minerals, are a testament to the fact that sometimes, the best beauty remedies are the simplest ones.

DIY Makeup: A Touch of Nature.

The realm of DIY doesn't end with skincare. Creating your own makeup, like a beetroot lip stain or cocoa powder bronzer, can be a delightful experience. These natural makeup products not only add beauty but also care for the skin, without the harsh chemicals found in commercial products.

The Power of Essential Oils.

Essential oils are nature's concentrated beauty elixirs. Adding a few drops of oils like lavender for soothing or tea tree for its antibacterial properties can transform a simple cream or lotion into a potent skin care remedy. It's about harnessing the natural potency of plants to care for our skin.

Mindful Beauty Routines.

Adopting a DIY approach to beauty is more than just about the products; it's about cultivating a mindful routine. Each step, from selecting ingredients to applying the product, is an act of self-care and a connection to nature. It's a journey that aligns with Barbara O'Neil's teachings of holistic health, where beauty is a reflection of overall well-being.

SUSTAINABLE PRACTICES IN BEAUTY.

DIY beauty is not just good for us but also for the planet. By choosing natural ingredients and creating products at home, we reduce the environmental impact of packaging and chemicals. It's a sustainable approach that respects the earth and our place within it.

THE JOY OF SHARING NATURAL BEAUTY.

The beauty of DIY natural beauty is that it can be shared. Creating products for friends and family, teaching them about the benefits of natural ingredients, is a way to spread the message of sustainable and healthy beauty practices. It's about building a community that values and respects the gifts of nature.

EMBRACING NATURE'S BEAUTY WISDOM.

The journey towards DIY natural beauty is a rewarding one, filled with discoveries and a deeper connection with nature. It's about returning to the basics, to the purity of ingredients that have cared for human beauty for centuries. This journey is not just about looking good; it's about feeling good and making choices that are in harmony with our bodies and the environment.

CREATIVE COOKING: DELICIOUS LEFTOVER IDEAS.

In our homes, we often find ourselves with an assortment of leftovers, sitting like forgotten treasures in the corners of our fridges. Today, I would like to take you on a delightful culinary journey, transforming these remnants into meals that tantalize the taste buds and warm the soul.

THE ART OF REPURPOSING LEFTOVERS.

The heart of creative cooking with leftovers lies in seeing the potential in what appears to be mundane. It's about blending traditional culinary wisdom with a modern twist. Think of a shepherd's pie using last night's roast and vegetables, or a hearty frittata enriched with bits of cheese and ham. It's these simple, ingenious combinations that make leftovers exciting again.

SOUP - A CANVAS FOR LEFTOVERS.

One of my favorite ways to utilize leftovers is in homemade soup. Nearly any combination of vegetables, grains, and proteins can be simmered into a nourishing broth. It's a method much in line with Barbara O'Neil's teachings of wholesome, holistic living - using what we have to nourish our bodies and reduce waste.

REVIVING DAY-OLD BREAD.

Stale bread is a common leftover that often gets discarded. However, it can be wonderfully repurposed. Think of French toast for a sweet start to the day, or savory croutons to add a crunch to your salads. Even making breadcrumbs for future recipes is a fantastic way to give old bread new life.

LEFTOVER VEGETABLES: A STIR-FRY DELIGHT.

Vegetables from last night can find new life in a stir-fry. A dash of soy sauce, a sprinkle of herbs, and a sizzle in the pan can transform them into a dish that's both tantalizing and nutritious. It's a perfect blend of ease and health, something Barbara O'Neil often advocates in her teachings on natural living.

REINVENTING PASTA AND RICE.

Leftover pasta or rice can be the base for a new creation. Turn rice into a delicious fried rice dish, or mix pasta with some fresh vegetables and a light dressing for a quick pasta salad. These simple yet effective ideas are not only practical but also align with a sustainable approach to food.

THE JOY OF BAKING WITH LEFTOVERS.

Baking with leftovers can be a delightful experiment. Overripe fruits become the stars in banana bread or fruit crumbles. Even leftover cooked vegetables can be incorporated into savory muffins or bread, creating a tasty and healthy treat.

WRAPS AND SANDWICHES: QUICK FIXES.

Wraps and sandwiches are perfect for using various leftovers in a new and exciting way. Fill them with last night's grilled chicken, roasted veggies, a sprinkle of cheese, and a spread of your choice. It's a quick, nutritious meal that encapsulates the essence of resourceful cooking.

PRESERVING AND PICKLING: A NOD TO TRADITION.

Preserving and pickling are age-old techniques that can be applied to leftovers, particularly fruits and vegetables. It's a method that connects us to the past while ensuring that nothing goes to waste. Pickled vegetables or homemade jams can add a burst of flavor to meals and are staples of a resourceful kitchen.

Leftover Grains: A Breakfast Twist.

Leftover grains like oatmeal or quinoa can be repurposed into nutritious breakfast options. Add some milk, a drizzle of honey, fresh fruits, and nuts, and you have a wholesome breakfast bowl. It's a testament to the versatility of simple ingredients and the power of a creative mind.

The Ethics of Leftover Cooking.

Cooking with leftovers also speaks to a deeper ethic of respect for our resources. It's about embracing a sustainable lifestyle, reducing food waste, and valuing what we have. This approach to cooking not only benefits our health but also our planet.

Embracing the Leftover Challenge.

Cooking with leftovers is an art form that invites creativity and resourcefulness. It's a practice that's both enjoyable and deeply satisfying, nourishing both the body and the soul. Each leftover ingredient is an opportunity to create something new, to experiment, and to enjoy the simple pleasures of home cooking.

WELLNESS IN PERSONAL GROWTH: SMALL STEPS, BIG GAINS.

In our journey through life, personal growth and wellness often go hand in hand. It's a symbiotic relationship where one feeds into the other, creating a harmonious balance. Embracing wellness in personal development is akin to nurturing a garden; it requires patience, care, and above all, an understanding that small steps lead to significant gains.

THE POWER OF INCREMENTAL CHANGE.

One of the most remarkable aspects of personal growth is the power of incremental change. Just as a stream carves a canyon over millennia, small, consistent efforts in our daily lives can lead to profound transformations. It's about cherishing the journey, not just the destination.

NURTURING MIND AND BODY.

The mind and body are intrinsically linked, and nurturing both is crucial for personal growth. Practices like yoga and meditation not only enhance physical flexibility and strength but also bring mental clarity and peace.

THE ROLE OF NUTRITION IN PERSONAL GROWTH.

Proper nutrition plays a pivotal role in personal development. Nourishing the body with wholesome foods is akin to fueling a vehicle with the right type of gas. It's about choosing foods that not only satisfy hunger but also provide the nutrients needed for mental and physical vigor.

Learning as a Wellness Practice.

The pursuit of knowledge and skills is a vital aspect of personal growth. Keep the mind active and engaged, whether through reading, taking up a new hobby, or even learning a new language. This continuous process of learning not only enriches our lives but also keeps our minds sharp and resilient.

The Power of Connection.

Human connections are at the heart of personal growth. Building and maintaining relationships, be they familial, platonic, or romantic, contribute to our sense of well-being. It's about cultivating a supportive network that encourages and sustains us through life's journey.

Physical Activity: A Pillar of Growth.

Regular physical activity is another cornerstone of personal development. It's not about rigorous gym sessions or intense workouts but finding joy in movement. A brisk walk, a leisurely bike ride, or a dance class can invigorate the body and elevate the mood.

Embracing Nature's Rhythms.

Aligning with nature's rhythms can profoundly impact our personal growth. It's about recognizing and respecting the natural cycles of waking and sleeping, activity and rest. This harmony with nature stresses the importance of living in sync with the natural world.

The Art of Mindfulness.

Mindfulness, the practice of being fully present in the moment, is a powerful tool for personal growth. It's about experiencing life as it unfolds, without judgment or distraction. This practice can be as simple as savoring a meal, enjoying a conversation, or observing the natural world with curiosity and wonder.

THE JOURNEY OF GROWTH.

Personal growth is a journey of small steps leading to significant gains. It is marked by the nurturing of mind and body, the pursuit of knowledge, the joy of physical movement, and the richness of human connections. By integrating these principles into our daily lives, we can achieve a state of wellness that not only enriches our own lives but also the lives of those around us.

BOOSTING ENERGY NATURALLY WITHOUT CAFFEINE.

In a world where the aroma of coffee seems to power our mornings and push us through our afternoons, the idea of boosting energy without caffeine might seem almost revolutionary. Yet, as we peel back the layers of traditional wisdom and modern understanding, we find a plethora of ways to invigorate our bodies and minds naturally. Let's consider these gentle, caffeine-free boosters, drawing inspiration from the teachings of natural health advocates like Barbara O'Neil.

THE SUNSHINE VITAMIN.

One of the simplest ways to enhance our energy levels is to step outside and bask in the morning sunshine. Vitamin D, often called the sunshine vitamin, plays a crucial role in energy metabolism. A brisk morning walk or a few minutes spent in a sunlit garden can do wonders for our spirit and vigor.

HYDRATION: THE ESSENCE OF VITALITY.

Often, fatigue is simply a sign of dehydration. Before reaching for a cup of coffee, try a glass of water. Infuse it with slices of lemon, cucumber, or mint for an extra refreshing twist. Hydration aids in digestion, circulation, and maintaining optimal bodily functions, which in turn keeps our energy levels steady.

BALANCED DIET: FUEL FOR THE DAY.

In the absence of caffeine, a well-balanced diet becomes our primary energy source. Focus on whole grains, lean proteins, and a variety of fruits and vegetables. Foods like bananas, apples, almonds, and oats provide sustained energy release, unlike the fleeting rush provided by caffeine.

Power Naps: A Rejuvenating Pause.

Sometimes, all it takes to recharge our batteries is a short power nap. A 20-minute rest can significantly improve alertness and performance without the need for caffeine. It's a technique often overlooked in our fast-paced society but one that offers profound restorative benefits.

Regular Exercise: Activating Natural Energy.

Regular physical activity, be it yoga, walking, or cycling, enhances our overall energy levels and mood. Exercise increases blood flow, improves sleep quality, and boosts endorphin levels, all of which contribute to a natural sense of vitality.

Mindful Breathing: Oxygenate Your Brain.

Mindful breathing exercises are a quick and effective way to energize the body. Deep, diaphragmatic breathing increases oxygen flow to the brain, reducing fatigue and foggy thinking. Even a few minutes of focused breathing can elevate energy levels.

Adaptogens: Nature's Stress Relievers.

Adaptogenic herbs like ashwagandha, rhodiola, and ginseng help in balancing the body's response to stress, a common energy drainer. Integrating these herbs into your diet can enhance physical stamina and mental clarity.

Laughter: The Best Medicine.

Never underestimate the power of laughter in boosting your energy. Laughter decreases stress hormones and increases endorphins. A good laugh can lighten your mood and invigorate your spirit.

SOCIAL CONNECTIONS: ENERGIZING RELATIONSHIPS.

Engaging in meaningful conversations and spending quality time with loved ones can also provide a significant energy boost. Positive social interactions stimulate the production of oxytocin, a hormone that has an energizing effect on our mood and overall well-being.

RESTORATIVE SLEEP: FOUNDATION OF ENERGY.

Finally, ensuring adequate, quality sleep is paramount in maintaining high energy levels. Establishing a relaxing bedtime routine and creating a sleep-conducive environment are essential steps in achieving restorative sleep.

EMBRACING NATURAL VITALITY.

Boosting energy naturally without caffeine is not only possible but also beneficial for our overall health. When we nurture our bodies with the right nutrients, engage in physical activity, and foster positive mental practices, we can sustain our energy levels throughout the day. These natural methods, inspired by traditional wisdom and validated by modern understanding, offer a harmonious approach to vitality and wellness.

Innovative Natural Remedies for Digestive Health.

The digestive system plays a central role, often referred to as the 'second brain' of our bodies. Today, let's discover some innovative natural remedies that can bolster our digestive health, weaving together traditional wisdom and a touch of modern understanding.

Fermented Foods: A Time-Honored Tradition.

The art of fermentation is as old as civilization itself. Foods like kefir, sauerkraut, kimchi, and miso are not only delightful to the taste buds but also teeming with probiotics. These beneficial bacteria are champions in enhancing gut flora, aiding digestion, and boosting immunity.

Herbal Teas: Nature's Soothing Elixir.

Herbal teas have been a staple in traditional medicine for centuries. Peppermint tea, for instance, is known for its ability to relieve bloating and improve digestion. Similarly, ginger tea can ease nausea and promote gastric mobility. Sipping these gentle brews can be both calming and beneficial for digestive health.

Chia Seeds: The Tiny Powerhouses.

Rich in fiber, omega-3 fatty acids, and antioxidants, chia seeds are a superb addition to a gut-friendly diet. When soaked, they form a gel-like substance that can aid in bowel regularity and promote a healthy gut.

Bone Broth: A Healing Tradition.

Bone broth, a rich source of minerals and amino acids, has been revered for generations for its gut-healing properties. It is believed to help in repairing gut lining and reducing inflammation, thereby aiding digestion.

Mindful Eating: The Art of Awareness.

Sometimes, the key to better digestion lies not just in what we eat but in how we eat. Mindful eating involves savoring each bite, chewing thoroughly, and listening to our body's cues. This practice not only enhances the digestive process but also deepens our connection with food.

Aloe Vera: More Than Just a Burn Remedy.

While known for its skin-soothing properties, aloe vera is also a potent digestive aid. Its anti-inflammatory and laxative properties can help soothe irritable bowel syndrome (IBS) symptoms and promote regularity.

Exercise: Stimulating Digestive Efficiency.

Regular exercise is crucial for maintaining digestive health. Physical activity helps stimulate the intestinal muscles, ensuring efficient movement of food through the digestive tract. Even a simple walk after meals can significantly aid digestion.

Hydration: The Foundation of Digestive Health.

Adequate hydration is essential for digestion. Water helps dissolve fats and soluble fiber, allowing these substances to pass through the intestines more easily. Herbal infusions and lemon water can be enjoyable ways to increase our water intake.

STRESS MANAGEMENT: CALMING THE DIGESTIVE NERVES.

Stress has a direct impact on our digestive system. Practices like yoga, meditation, and deep breathing can reduce stress levels, thereby improving our digestive health. Taking time to relax and unwind is not just good for the mind, but also for the gut.

EMBRACING HOLISTIC PRACTICES.

Incorporating these practices into our daily lives nurtures our digestive system, which in turn enhances our overall well-being. From savoring fermented foods to practicing mindful eating, each step we take is a stride towards better health. These remedies, rooted in traditional wisdom and complemented by modern insights, offer us a harmonious path to digestive wellness.

FITNESS AT HOME: EASY AND EFFECTIVE EXERCISES.

The pursuit of fitness and well-being continues, unfazed by the bustling world outside. Today, I invite you to examine simple yet effective home exercises that seamlessly blend traditional wisdom with modern understanding.

BODYWEIGHT EXERCISES: THE FOUNDATION OF HOME FITNESS.

The beauty of bodyweight exercises lies in their simplicity and effectiveness. Push-ups, for instance, are a timeless classic that strengthens the chest, arms, and core. For beginners, wall or knee push-ups offer a gentle start. Then, there are squats and lunges, perfect for toning legs and glutes while improving balance.

YOGA: A DANCE OF STRENGTH AND FLEXIBILITY.

Yoga, an ancient practice with roots in holistic well-being, is perfect for a home workout. Simple poses like the downward dog or the warrior series not only improve flexibility but also build strength. Incorporating yoga into daily routines creates a space for mindfulness amidst physical activity.

PILATES: CORE AND MORE.

Pilates, a form of exercise focusing on core strength, postural alignment, and muscle balance, is wonderfully adaptable to home environments. Exercises like the plank, leg circles, and the hundred can be done with minimal space and equipment, yet they offer profound benefits in flexibility and strength.

RESISTANCE BANDS: A VERSATILE TOOL.

Resistance bands are a fantastic addition to home workouts. They add variety and intensity to exercises like bicep curls, tricep extensions, and leg presses. Plus, they're lightweight and portable, ideal for small spaces.

CARDIOVASCULAR FITNESS: GETTING THE HEART PUMPING.

For cardiovascular health, nothing beats a good heart-pumping session. Jumping jacks, brisk walking in place, or even dancing to your favorite tunes can elevate the heart rate effectively. Remember, it's about moving more and sitting less.

BALANCE EXERCISES: A KEY TO GRACEFUL AGING.

As Barbara O'Neil often emphasizes, maintaining balance is crucial, especially as we age. Simple exercises like standing on one foot or walking heel to toe can significantly improve balance and coordination.

STRETCHING: THE ART OF FLEXIBILITY.

Stretching is an integral part of any fitness routine, offering benefits like improved flexibility and reduced muscle tension. Gentle stretches in the morning or after a workout can be incredibly rejuvenating.

MINDFUL MOVEMENTS: THE CONNECTION BETWEEN BODY AND MIND.

Incorporating mindfulness into our fitness regime enhances the connection between body and mind. Exercises like tai chi or qigong, with their fluid, deliberate movements, are not only physically beneficial but also mentally soothing.

HYDRATION AND NUTRITION: FUELING THE BODY NATURALLY.

As we engage in physical activities, proper hydration and nutrition become paramount. Sipping herbal teas or water infused with lemon and mint, and consuming a balanced diet rich in fruits, vegetables, and whole grains support our fitness journey.

EMBRACING HOLISTIC HOME FITNESS.

Fitness at home is a journey that blends simplicity with effectiveness. Whether it's through the strength of bodyweight exercises, the flexibility of yoga, or the rhythm of cardiovascular workouts, each step we take is a stride towards holistic health. We must cherish this journey, infusing our daily routines with these nurturing practices, and witness the transformative power of home fitness.

Ergonomic Living: Comfort in Everyday Spaces.

The way we interact with our environment significantly impacts our well-being. I, am here to guide you through the art of ergonomic living; a blend of traditional wisdom and modern understanding, to learn how simple changes in our everyday spaces can bring comfort and improve our overall health.

Understanding Ergonomics: More Than Just Comfort.

Ergonomics isn't just about being comfortable; it's about creating environments that support our body's natural posture and movements. This concept, deeply rooted in the understanding of human anatomy, aligns perfectly with traditional practices that emphasize harmony with nature.

The Ergonomic Home Office: A Necessity, Not a Luxury.

With many of us spending hours in home offices, ergonomic design is crucial. Start with your chair: it should support your lower back and encourage a straight, yet relaxed posture. Your computer screen should be at eye level to avoid neck strain. Barbara O'Neil often spoke about the importance of natural elements; consider placing plants in your office space to enhance air quality and mood.

The Kitchen: Cooking with Ease.

The kitchen, often the heart of the home, can be a place of ergonomic joy. Organize your space so that frequently used items are within easy reach. When designing your kitchen, consider counter heights that prevent stooping or stretching and flooring that cushions your feet during long cooking sessions.

LIVING SPACES: RELAXATION AND MOVEMENT.

In our living areas, furniture should support a comfortable yet active posture. Avoid overly soft couches that cause slouching. Choose seating that allows your feet to rest flat on the floor, with knees at a right angle. Incorporate spaces for movement or stretching, a concept Barbara O'Neil frequently advocated for overall health.

BEDROOMS: A HAVEN FOR RESTORATIVE SLEEP.

The bedroom should be a sanctuary for restorative sleep. Choose a mattress and pillows that support your natural spinal alignment. The idea is to create a space that promotes relaxation and rejuvenation, in line with holistic wellness principles.

BATHROOMS: SAFETY AND ACCESSIBILITY.

In the bathroom, consider non-slip mats and adequate lighting to prevent accidents. Ergonomic designs like raised toilet seats or walk-in showers can be particularly beneficial for those with limited mobility.

LIGHTING: THE NATURAL ENERGY BOOSTER.

Proper lighting is essential for an ergonomic home. Natural light is best, so open those curtains wide! For artificial lighting, choose sources that reduce glare and eye strain. Barbara O'Neil's teachings on the importance of sunlight in health remind us of the vitality that natural light brings to our spaces.

Gardens and Outdoor Spaces: Blending Function and Nature.

For those with gardens or balconies, ergonomic design can create a delightful and functional outdoor space. Raised beds or container gardens can reduce bending and stooping, making gardening a joy rather than a chore.

Ergonomic Living for a Healthier You.

Ergonomic living entails creating spaces that not only comfort but also enhance our well-being. It's about understanding our interaction with our surroundings and making adjustments that support our health. When we incorporate these simple yet effective ergonomic principles into our daily lives, we not only create a more comfortable living environment but also embrace a lifestyle that fosters health and well-being.

Healthy Snacking: Guilt-Free Treats.

The concept of snacking often comes with a hint of guilt. Still, snacking can indeed be a delightful, guilt-free experience. We will look into the world of healthy snacking, where nourishment meets taste.

The Philosophy of Healthy Snacking.

Healthy snacking isn't just about choosing the right foods; it's a mindset. It's about finding a balance between indulgence and nutrition. Snacking should satisfy not just the taste buds but also contribute to your overall well-being.

Understanding Hunger and Fullness.

Before reaching for a snack, it's important to tune in to your body's signals. Are you truly hungry, or is it boredom or emotion driving you to eat? Listening to your body's natural hunger cues is a practice often emphasized in natural health teachings.

The Art of Choosing Your Snacks.

The key to guilt-free snacking lies in the choices you make. Opt for whole, unprocessed foods. Think fruits, nuts, seeds, and whole grains. These natural foods, are not only nutritious but also provide the energy boost you need.

Fruits: Nature's Sweet Treats.

Fruits are nature's candy. Full of vitamins, minerals, and fiber, they are the perfect snack. Try apple slices with almond butter, a small bowl of berries, or a banana for a quick, satisfying treat.

NUTS AND SEEDS: NUTRIENT-DENSE SNACKS.

Nuts and seeds are little powerhouses of nutrients. A small handful of almonds, walnuts, or pumpkin seeds can provide a satisfying crunch along with healthy fats, proteins, and fiber.

VEGETABLES: CRISP AND REFRESHING.

Vegetables aren't just for meals. Carrot sticks, cucumber slices, or cherry tomatoes can be a refreshing snack. Pair them with hummus or guacamole for added flavor and nutrients.

WHOLE GRAINS: SUSTAINED ENERGY.

Whole grains provide sustained energy. A small serving of oatmeal, whole-grain crackers, or popcorn can be both satisfying and healthful. Remember, portion control is key!

HEALTHY DIPS AND SPREADS.

Dips and spreads can turn simple fruits, vegetables, or grains into a delightful snack. Try making your own dips with yogurt, herbs, or avocados for a healthier alternative to store-bought options.

HYDRATION: AN IMPORTANT PART OF SNACKING.

Often, we mistake thirst for hunger. Staying well-hydrated is crucial. Herbal teas, water infused with fruits, or simply plain water can be refreshing companions to your snacks.

MINDFUL SNACKING: ENJOY EVERY BITE.

Mindful eating is a concept often embraced in holistic health. Savor each bite, chew slowly, and enjoy the flavors and textures. This not only enhances the snacking experience but also helps in better digestion and satisfaction.

SNACKING AND MEAL BALANCE.

Healthy snacking should complement your meals, not replace them. Plan your snacks to fit into your overall diet, ensuring a balance of carbohydrates, proteins, and fats throughout the day.

HOMEMADE SNACKS: THE JOY OF CREATING.

There's joy and health in homemade snacks. Simple recipes like roasted chickpeas, homemade granola bars, or fruit and nut balls can be both fun to make and nourishing.

EMBRACE THE JOY OF HEALTHY SNACKING.

Snacking can indeed be a healthy and enjoyable part of your day. By choosing the right foods and embracing the principles of mindful eating, you can indulge in guilt-free treats that nourish and satisfy. Healthy snacking is not just about the food; it's a delightful journey towards wellness.

MINDFUL MOVEMENT: INTEGRATING FITNESS INTO DAILY LIFE.

Finding time for fitness can be challenging. Yet, integrating movement into our daily routine can be both enriching and attainable. Let's see how mindful movement can be seamlessly woven into the fabric of our everyday lives.

THE ESSENCE OF MINDFUL MOVEMENT.

Mindful movement is about being present and aware during physical activity. It's not just about the body moving, but also about the mind engaging with and appreciating each movement. This approach aligns beautifully with Barbara O'Neil's teachings, which emphasize the connection between mind, body, and spirit.

STARTING WITH SMALL STEPS.

The journey towards incorporating fitness into daily life can begin with the simplest of actions. It might be taking the stairs instead of the elevator, walking to the local store rather than driving, or even standing while talking on the phone. These small choices add up, creating a foundation for a more active lifestyle.

STRETCHING: A SIMPLE YET POWERFUL TOOL.

Stretching is a wonderfully accessible form of exercise that can be done anywhere and at any time. Whether it's a morning stretch to awaken the body or a few minutes of stretching at your desk to relieve tension, this practice can significantly improve flexibility, circulation, and overall well-being.

Walking: The Underrated Exercise.

Walking is often underestimated, yet it is one of the most natural forms of exercise. A brisk walk in the park, a leisurely stroll in the evening, or even pacing while on a phone call are excellent ways to keep the body moving. Walking not only benefits physical health but also clears the mind.

Incorporating Movement into Household Chores.

Household chores can be a surprising source of physical activity. Gardening, cleaning, or even cooking can be transformed into opportunities for fitness. Performing these tasks with mindfulness and vigor can turn mundane activities into enjoyable exercise.

Yoga and Pilates: Strengthening and Toning.

Yoga and Pilates can be easily integrated into daily life. These practices strengthen and tone the body while also enhancing flexibility. Even a short session in the morning or evening can have profound effects on physical and mental health.

Dance: Joyful Expression through Movement.

Dancing is not only fun but also an excellent way to exercise. Putting on your favorite music and dancing around the living room can elevate your heart rate and lift your spirits, embodying the holistic approach to health.

Breathing Exercises: Enhancing Movement with Breath.

Breathing exercises are a key component of mindful movement. Conscious breathing during exercise improves oxygen flow, enhances performance, and helps in centering the mind, aligning with the principles of natural health.

BALANCE AND COORDINATION EXERCISES.

Simple balance and coordination exercises can be done at home with little to no equipment. Practices like standing on one leg or using balance balls can improve core strength and stability, which are crucial for overall health and well-being.

MINDFUL MOVEMENT IN THE WORKPLACE.

Incorporating movement into your workday can have significant benefits. Simple actions like taking walking meetings, using a standing desk, or performing chair exercises can counteract the negative effects of prolonged sitting.

TECHNOLOGY AND FITNESS: HARNESSING THE DIGITAL AGE.

Technology, when used mindfully, can be a great ally in integrating fitness into daily life. Fitness apps, online exercise programs, and even virtual trainers can provide guidance and motivation right in the comfort of your home.

SETTING REALISTIC GOALS.

It's important to set achievable fitness goals. Whether it's walking a certain number of steps each day, stretching every morning, or practicing yoga twice a week, these goals should be realistic and tailored to fit into your lifestyle.

THE JOY OF OUTDOOR ACTIVITIES.

Engaging in outdoor activities like hiking, cycling, or even playing sports can be a delightful way to incorporate exercise into your routine. These activities not only provide physical benefits but also allow you to connect with nature, a concept often emphasized in natural health teachings.

COMMUNITY INVOLVEMENT: GROUP FITNESS AND SOCIAL INTERACTION.

Participating in group fitness classes or community sports can add a social dimension to exercise. These activities not only improve physical health but also promote social well-being, resonating with Barbara O'Neil's holistic view of health.

EMBRACING FITNESS AS A LIFESTYLE.

Taking fitness as a daily lifestyle doesn't have to be a daunting task. Making mindful movement and small, consistent changes will significantly enhance our physical and mental well-being.

Wholesome Breakfast Ideas for a Healthy Start.

Starting the day with a nourishing breakfast sets the tone for what's to come. I firmly believe in the power of a wholesome morning meal to energize the body, soothe the mind, and align with nature's wisdom. Let's find some delightful breakfast ideas that blend traditional wisdom, akin to Barbara O'Neil's teachings, with a touch of modern practicality.

The Foundation of a Wholesome Breakfast.

A wholesome breakfast is more than just a meal; it's a celebration of nature's bounty. It should be balanced, including a mix of complex carbohydrates, healthy fats, and proteins. These elements ensure sustained energy levels throughout the morning.

Oatmeal: A Timeless Classic.

Oatmeal is a versatile and hearty option. For a nutrient-packed breakfast, cook oats in almond milk and top them with fresh fruits, nuts, and a drizzle of honey. This dish is not only delicious but also rich in fiber and essential nutrients.

Smoothie Bowls: Nutrition Meets Creativity.

Smoothie bowls are a fantastic way to pack a variety of nutrients into one meal. Blend your favorite fruits with Greek yogurt or plant-based milk, pour it into a bowl, and top with seeds, nuts, and granola. This is a delightful way to enjoy a colorful, antioxidant-rich breakfast.

Wholegrain Toast: Simple Yet Satisfying.

Wholegrain toast can be the base for numerous healthy toppings. Avocado with poached eggs, almond butter with banana slices, or cottage cheese with berries are all excellent choices. Each provides a good balance of macronutrients and keeps you full for longer.

Homemade Granola: Crunchy Delight.

Making your granola allows you to control the ingredients and sugar content. Mix oats, nuts, seeds, and dried fruits, then bake with a touch of maple syrup and coconut oil. Serve with yogurt or milk for a crunchy, fiber-rich breakfast.

Chia Pudding: A Modern Twist.

Chia seeds soaked overnight in almond milk create a pudding-like consistency, ideal for a light yet filling breakfast. Add a layer of fruit puree or compote, and top with fresh fruits for a delightful and nutritious start to your day.

Egg-Based Dishes: Protein-Packed Start.

Eggs are a wonderful source of protein. An omelet with spinach, tomatoes, and feta, or scrambled eggs with herbs and avocado, are both excellent ways to incorporate vegetables and protein into your first meal.

Savory Porridge: A Heartier Option.

Not all porridge needs to be sweet. A savory porridge with quinoa or millet, seasoned with herbs and topped with a poached egg or sautéed vegetables, can be a comforting and satisfying breakfast.

Fruit and Yogurt Parfait: Layers of Goodness.

Layer Greek yogurt with fruits, nuts, and a drizzle of honey or maple syrup in a glass. This not only looks appealing but is a great combination of probiotics, vitamins, and minerals.

Pancakes with a Twist.

Whip up pancakes using whole wheat or oat flour and add mashed bananas or applesauce for natural sweetness. Serve with fresh fruits and a dollop of yogurt for a delightful breakfast.

Breakfast Wraps: A Convenient Choice.

For those on the go, breakfast wraps are perfect. Fill a whole-grain wrap with scrambled eggs, avocado, and salsa or with peanut butter, banana, and granola for a quick, portable meal.

Nut and Seed Bread: A Hearty Alternative.

Baking your bread with nuts, seeds, and whole grains can be a fulfilling project. This type of bread is not only delicious but also packed with nutrients and makes for an excellent breakfast base.

Tea or Herbal Infusions: A Soothing Start.

Starting the day with a warm cup of tea or a herbal infusion can be calming. Whether it's green tea, chamomile, or a homemade blend, this ritual complements a nutritious breakfast beautifully.

The Importance of Mindfulness.

Remember, a wholesome breakfast is not just about the food, but also about the experience. Eating mindfully, savoring each bite, and being present in the moment enhances the nutritional benefits and aligns with the holistic approach to health.

A Day Begins with Breakfast.

A wholesome breakfast is key to a healthy, energetic start to the day. By combining traditional wisdom with modern understanding, we can create breakfasts that are not only nutritious but also a joy to eat.

Lunch Recipes for Sustained Energy.

Lunch, the midday meal, is a critical part of our daily nutrition. It's a moment to refuel and re-energize our bodies for the afternoon ahead. The key is to choose ingredients that provide sustained energy and incorporate them into delightful and nourishing recipes. These lunch ideas draw inspiration from traditional wisdom, with a nod to modern dietary understanding, perhaps echoing the holistic approach of Barbara O'Neil.

Quinoa and Black Bean Salad: A Protein Powerhouse.

Quinoa, a complete protein, pairs beautifully with fiber-rich black beans in this salad. Toss with chopped tomatoes, avocado, fresh cilantro, and a lime dressing for a refreshing yet filling meal. This salad provides a perfect balance of protein, fiber, and healthy fats.

Hearty Vegetable Soup: Comfort in a Bowl.

A vegetable soup with lentils or chickpeas is warming and satisfying. Add a variety of seasonal vegetables, some herbs, and spices for flavor, and let it simmer to perfection. This soup is a comforting dish that nourishes the body and soul.

Whole Wheat Pasta with Pesto and Roasted Vegetables.

Whole wheat pasta offers more fiber and nutrients than its white counterpart. Toss it with homemade pesto and a medley of roasted vegetables for a meal that's both hearty and healthy. It's a simple yet delicious way to incorporate more vegetables into the diet.

MEDITERRANEAN CHICKPEA WRAPS: A TASTE OF THE MIDDLE EAST.

Fill whole-grain wraps with chickpeas, cucumbers, tomatoes, olives, and feta cheese. Drizzle with a tahini-lemon sauce for a Mediterranean-inspired lunch. This wrap is not only tasty but also provides a good balance of nutrients.

BUDDHA BOWL: A BIT OF EVERYTHING.

A Buddha bowl is a great way to enjoy a variety of nutrients in one meal. Start with a base of brown rice or mixed greens, add a protein like grilled tofu or chicken, and top with an assortment of vegetables. Finish with a drizzle of a healthy dressing for a colorful and balanced meal.

STUFFED SWEET POTATOES: A SWEET AND SAVORY TREAT.

Bake sweet potatoes and stuff them with a mix of quinoa, black beans, corn, and bell peppers. Top with avocado and a dollop of Greek yogurt for a meal that's as satisfying as it is nutritious. Sweet potatoes are an excellent source of vitamins and fiber.

AVOCADO AND EGG SALAD SANDWICH: A CREAMY DELIGHT.

Mash avocado with hard-boiled eggs, add a bit of mustard, and season to taste. Spread on whole-grain bread for a twist on the classic egg salad sandwich. This meal is rich in protein and healthy fats, keeping you full and energized.

ASIAN-INSPIRED CHICKEN LETTUCE WRAPS.

Cook minced chicken with garlic, ginger, and soy sauce. Serve in lettuce cups and top with shredded carrots, bean sprouts, and a sprinkle of sesame seeds. These wraps are light yet flavorful, providing a good balance of protein and fresh vegetables.

GRILLED SALMON WITH QUINOA AND STEAMED GREENS.

Grill a salmon fillet and serve it with quinoa and a side of steamed greens like kale or spinach. Salmon is rich in omega-3 fatty acids, which are beneficial for heart and brain health.

TURMERIC RICE WITH VEGETABLES AND LENTILS.

Cook rice with turmeric, a spice known for its anti-inflammatory properties. Mix in cooked lentils and sautéed vegetables for a simple yet nutrient-dense meal. This dish is comforting and packed with health benefits.

A MIDDAY MEAL TO ENERGIZE AND SUSTAIN.

Using these recipes in the lunch routine can help maintain energy levels throughout the day. By choosing ingredients that offer sustained energy and preparing them in ways that are both nourishing and enjoyable, lunch can become a delightful and energizing part of the day. As with any dietary advice, it's always recommended to listen to the body and adjust according to personal health needs and preferences.

DINNER IDEAS: NOURISHING AND DELICIOUS.

Dinner is not just a meal; it's a time to gather, to nourish, and to reflect on the day. It's an opportunity to feed both the body and soul with flavors that inspire and ingredients that heal. The dinner recipes here focus on wholesome, natural ingredients that are as delightful to the palate as they are beneficial to health.

ROASTED VEGETABLE AND CHICKPEA BOWL.

Roasting brings out the natural sweetness and depth of flavor in vegetables. Combine roasted carrots, broccoli, and red peppers with chickpeas for a protein-rich base. Serve over brown rice or quinoa and drizzle with a lemon-tahini sauce. This bowl is a symphony of flavors and nutrients.

HERB-INFUSED GRILLED CHICKEN WITH STEAMED GREENS.

Marinate chicken breasts in a blend of fresh herbs, olive oil, and garlic. Grill to perfection and serve with a side of steamed green vegetables like spinach or kale. This dish is simple, packed with protein, and enriched with the healing power of herbs.

LENTIL AND MUSHROOM STEW.

Lentils are a wonderful source of plant-based protein and fiber. Cook them with mushrooms, onions, carrots, and a rich tomato base for a hearty stew. Serve with a slice of whole-grain bread for a comforting, filling meal.

BAKED SALMON WITH ASPARAGUS AND QUINOA SALAD.

Salmon, a fantastic source of omega-3 fatty acids, pairs well with asparagus and a lemony quinoa salad. This meal is light yet satisfying, perfect for an evening of relaxation and rejuvenation.

VEGETABLE STIR-FRY WITH TOFU AND BROWN RICE.

A stir-fry is a quick, versatile dinner option. Use a variety of colorful vegetables and firm tofu for a protein punch. Serve over brown rice, which provides more fiber and nutrients than white rice. A splash of soy sauce and a hint of ginger add an Asian twist to this dish.

SWEET POTATO AND BLACK BEAN ENCHILADAS.

Wrap a mixture of mashed sweet potatoes and black beans in corn tortillas. Top with a homemade tomato sauce and bake until bubbly. This dish is a delightful blend of sweet and savory flavors, rich in fiber and plant-based protein.

MEDITERRANEAN-STYLE STUFFED PEPPERS.

Stuff bell peppers with a mixture of quinoa, chopped tomatoes, olives, and feta cheese. Bake until the peppers are tender and the filling is warm. This meal is not only visually appealing but also packed with flavors of the Mediterranean.

SPAGHETTI SQUASH WITH PESTO AND ROASTED TOMATOES.

Spaghetti squash is a wonderful low-carb alternative to pasta. Roast it and scrape out the strands, then mix with homemade pesto and roasted cherry tomatoes. This dish is light, flavorful, and nourishing.

CURRIED CAULIFLOWER AND CHICKPEA CASSEROLE.

Combine cauliflower, chickpeas, and peas in a coconut milk and curry sauce. Bake until golden and bubbly. This casserole is a fusion of flavors, comforting and rich in spices that aid digestion and boost health.

ZUCCHINI NOODLES WITH AVOCADO PESTO AND CHERRY TOMATOES.

For a light and refreshing dinner, spiralize zucchinis into noodles and toss with a creamy avocado pesto. Add cherry tomatoes for a pop of color and sweetness. This dish is wonderfully satisfying, yet surprisingly light.

A FEAST FOR HEALTH AND PLEASURE.

These dinner ideas showcase how easy and enjoyable it is to incorporate healthful, natural ingredients into the evening meal. Each recipe is crafted to maximize both nutritional value and flavor, ensuring that dinner is not only a time to satiate hunger but also to celebrate health and wellness. The key to a nourishing dinner lies in the quality of ingredients and the joy of sharing it with loved ones.

HEALTHY DESSERTS: GUILT-FREE INDULGENCES.

Desserts often carry a reputation for being a guilty pleasure, but they can be transformed into wholesome treats that nourish as much as they delight. The secret lies in using natural, healthful ingredients and a bit of creativity. Here are some delightful dessert ideas that allow indulgence without the guilt.

1. Avocado Chocolate Mousse.

Creamy, rich, and utterly satisfying, this mousse uses ripe avocados for a silky texture and heart-healthy fats. Blend avocados with cocoa powder, a touch of maple syrup, and vanilla extract for a luscious dessert. It's a perfect example of how natural ingredients can create something decadently delicious.

2. Baked Apples with Cinnamon and Nuts.

Simple yet utterly comforting, baked apples are a treat that harkens back to simpler times. Core some apples, fill them with a mix of nuts, cinnamon, and a drizzle of honey, then bake until tender. This dessert is a delightful blend of natural sweetness and warming spices.

3. Banana Ice Cream.

Frozen bananas can be transformed into a creamy and sweet ice cream without any added sugar. Simply blend frozen bananas until smooth. Add flavors like peanut butter, cocoa powder, or vanilla to enhance this simple treat. It's a fantastic way to use overripe bananas and get a dose of potassium.

4. Dark Chocolate-Dipped Strawberries.

Melt some high-quality dark chocolate, rich in antioxidants, and dip fresh strawberries into it. Once the chocolate sets, you have a delightful treat that's both luxurious and packed with nutrients. It's a classic combination that never fails to please.

5. Almond Flour Lemon Bars.

Using almond flour for the crust gives these lemon bars a nutritious twist. Top with a lemon curd made from fresh lemon juice, eggs, and a touch of honey. These bars are a tangy, sweet delight, offering a good dose of vitamin C and healthy fats.

6. Coconut Yogurt Parfait with Berries and Granola.

Layer coconut yogurt with fresh berries and homemade granola for a dessert that could double as a nutritious breakfast. The yogurt provides probiotics, the berries are full of antioxidants, and the granola adds a satisfying crunch.

7. Chia Seed Pudding.

Chia seeds soaked in almond milk become a pudding-like dessert that's high in omega-3 fatty acids and fiber. Sweeten with a bit of maple syrup and top with fresh fruit for a simple, healthful dessert that's also incredibly versatile.

8. Flourless Peanut Butter Cookies.

With just a few ingredients; peanut butter, an egg, and a natural sweetener like honey; you can create a batch of delicious cookies that are both satisfying and free of refined flour. They're a hit with kids and adults alike.

9. Oatmeal and Raisin Cookies with Apple Sauce..

Replacing sugar with apple sauce in oatmeal and raisin cookies not only reduces the calorie count but also adds a natural sweetness and moist texture. Add a sprinkle of cinnamon for a warm, comforting flavor.

10. Carrot Cake with Greek Yogurt Frosting.

A carrot cake made with whole wheat flour, natural sweeteners, and plenty of grated carrots, topped with a tangy Greek yogurt frosting, is a delightful way to enjoy dessert. It's a classic favorite with a healthier twist.

SWEETNESS WITHOUT THE SIN.

These healthy dessert ideas prove that satisfying a sweet tooth doesn't have to mean compromising on health. By using natural ingredients and making smart swaps, it's possible to enjoy delectable desserts that are not only guilt-free but also beneficial to overall wellness.

Natural Solutions for Healthy Skin.

The pursuit of healthy, radiant skin is often cluttered with complex skincare routines and expensive products. But sometimes, the most effective solutions are rooted in simplicity and nature. This section discusses natural skincare, blending traditional wisdom with modern understanding.

Understanding Skin Health.

Healthy skin starts with understanding its needs. Skin, the largest organ of the body, serves as a protective barrier and is a reflection of overall health. Factors like diet, hydration, sleep, and stress levels significantly impact skin health. Embracing a holistic approach to skincare means caring for the body both inside and out.

Hydration and Diet.

The foundation of healthy skin is proper hydration and a balanced diet. Drinking plenty of water and consuming a diet rich in fruits, vegetables, lean proteins, and healthy fats provides the skin with essential nutrients. Foods high in antioxidants, such as berries, nuts, and green leafy vegetables, combat free radicals and promote skin health.

Natural Cleansers.

Commercial cleansers often contain harsh chemicals that strip the skin of its natural oils. A gentler approach involves using natural ingredients like honey, known for its antibacterial properties, or oatmeal, which has soothing and anti-inflammatory effects. These natural cleansers help maintain the skin's pH balance and retain its natural moisture.

Exfoliation with Natural Ingredients.

Exfoliating is crucial for removing dead skin cells and revealing brighter skin. Natural exfoliants like sugar or coffee grounds mixed with olive oil can be effective and gentle alternatives to chemical exfoliants.

Moisturizing with Oils.

Natural oils like coconut, jojoba, and almond oil are excellent for moisturizing the skin. They are easily absorbed and mimic the skin's natural sebum, preventing dryness without clogging pores.

Sun Protection.

Sun exposure can cause premature aging and skin damage. Natural solutions like wearing protective clothing and using zinc oxide-based sunscreens can provide effective protection against harmful UV rays.

Soothing Inflammation with Aloe Vera.

Aloe vera is renowned for its soothing and healing properties. It's beneficial for treating sunburns, inflammation, and irritation. This plant can be used directly from the garden, emphasizing the simplicity of natural remedies.

Anti-Aging with Green Tea.

Green tea is packed with antioxidants, making it excellent for combating signs of aging. Applying green tea bags or a homemade green tea toner can reduce puffiness and improve skin elasticity.

Herbal Remedies.

Herbs like chamomile, lavender, and calendula have been used for centuries in skincare. They can be infused in oils or used as tea rinses to calm irritated skin and promote healing.

Stress Management for Skin Health.

Stress can wreak havoc on the skin, leading to issues like acne and eczema. Practices such as yoga, meditation, and sufficient rest are crucial for managing stress and maintaining healthy skin.

A Return to Nature.

Embracing natural skincare methods is not just about being trendy; it's about respecting and harnessing the power of nature for overall well-being. Making use of these simple yet effective natural solutions as a daily routine keeps achieving healthy, glowing skin within reach.

Travel Wellness: Staying Healthy on the Go.

Traveling opens doors to new experiences, cultures, and memories. Maintaining health while on the move can be a challenge. This section al and natural strategies to stay healthy, combining the wisdom of traditional practices with modern insights, reminiscent of Barbara O'Neil's teachings.

Pre-Travel Preparation.

A healthy journey begins even before leaving home. Boosting the immune system is key. A diet rich in fruits, vegetables, and probiotics prepares the body for the different environments it will encounter. Packing a small health kit with natural remedies like ginger for motion sickness, echinacea for immune support, and lavender oil for relaxation can be a lifesaver.

Hydration is Key.

Staying hydrated is crucial, especially when flying. The air in airplanes is notably dry, which can lead to dehydration. Carrying a reusable water bottle and sipping water throughout the journey helps maintain hydration levels. Herbal teas can be a comforting way to stay hydrated and calm.

Nutrition on the Go.

Finding healthy food options while traveling can be challenging. Packing nutritious snacks like nuts, fruits, and homemade granola bars ensures access to healthy options. When dining out, choosing meals with fresh ingredients and avoiding processed foods helps maintain a balanced diet.

Active Travel.

Incorporating physical activity into travel plans isn't just good for the body; it's a wonderful way to explore new places. Walking tours, hiking, swimming, or even morning stretches at the hotel can keep the body active and energized.

Rest and Sleep.

Travel can disrupt sleep patterns. Natural sleep aids like chamomile tea or valerian root can promote restful sleep. Practicing good sleep hygiene by keeping a regular sleep schedule and creating a calming pre-sleep routine can also help.

Mindfulness and Relaxation.

Travel can be stressful. Practicing mindfulness and relaxation techniques such as deep breathing, meditation, or yoga can reduce stress levels. These practices not only keep the mind calm but also enhance the travel experience by fostering a deeper connection with the surroundings.

Sun Protection.

Protecting the skin from the sun is essential, especially in unfamiliar climates. Wearing hats, sunglasses, and applying natural sunscreens protects the skin from harmful UV rays and prevents sunburn.

Avoiding Jet Lag.

Jet lag can be mitigated by adjusting sleep patterns a few days before the trip to align with the destination time zone. Staying hydrated and avoiding alcohol and caffeine during the flight also helps in reducing jet lag symptoms.

Safe and Clean.

In unfamiliar environments, it's important to be mindful of cleanliness. Carrying natural hand sanitizers and disinfectant wipes, and being cautious with water and food sources in areas with known health risks, are prudent practices.

Connecting with Nature.

Whenever possible, connecting with nature during travel can have a profound impact on health. Activities like forest bathing, beach walks, or simply spending time in a park can rejuvenate the mind and body.

Embracing Healthy Travel.

Traveling healthily is about balancing enjoyment with well-being. By planning ahead, making smart food choices, staying active, and taking time for relaxation and mindfulness, travelers can maintain their health and enhance their travel experience.

ECO-FRIENDLY HOME PRACTICES FOR HEALTH.

In a world where environmental concerns and personal well-being are increasingly intertwined, adopting eco-friendly home practices is not just a choice but a necessity. These practices, rooted in traditional wisdom and enhanced by modern understanding, offer a path to a healthier lifestyle and a thriving planet. We shall learn how simple, eco-friendly changes in our homes can lead to significant health benefits.

NATURAL CLEANING SOLUTIONS.

Chemical-laden cleaning products are not only harmful to the environment but also to our health. Switching to natural cleaning agents like vinegar, baking soda, and essential oils can reduce exposure to harmful chemicals. These natural alternatives are effective, affordable, and kinder to the planet.

INDOOR AIR QUALITY.

Indoor air quality is crucial for health. Plants are nature's air purifiers, removing toxins and improving air quality. Incorporating plants like spider plants, peace lilies, and aloe vera can enhance indoor air quality while adding a touch of greenery to your living space.

MINDFUL ENERGY CONSUMPTION.

Reducing energy consumption is key to eco-friendly living. Simple practices like using LED bulbs, unplugging devices when not in use, and maximizing natural light can significantly reduce energy use and contribute to a healthier environment.

Sustainable Eating Habits.

What we eat impacts not only our health but also the environment. Embracing a diet rich in organic, locally-sourced, and plant-based foods can reduce the ecological footprint. Growing your own herbs and vegetables, even in small spaces, can reconnect you with the process of food production and ensure a fresh, toxin-free supply.

Eco-Friendly Personal Care.

The personal care industry is notorious for its environmental impact. Opting for products with natural ingredients and eco-friendly packaging can reduce exposure to harmful substances and environmental harm. DIY personal care products, like homemade face masks or natural toothpaste, can be healthy, fun, and sustainable.

Mindful Water Usage.

Water is a precious resource. Practices like installing low-flow showerheads, fixing leaks, and using rainwater for gardening can significantly reduce water consumption.

Reducing Plastic Use.

Plastic pollution is a pressing environmental issue. Reducing plastic use by opting for reusable bags, containers, and eco-friendly materials helps minimize waste and protect marine life.

Sustainable Furnishing.

Choosing furniture made from sustainable materials, repurposing old items, and opting for second-hand or vintage pieces can reduce environmental impact and add a unique charm to your home.

Mindful Waste Management.

Effective waste management is crucial for an eco-friendly home. Composting organic waste, recycling, and repurposing items can significantly reduce the waste that ends up in landfills.

Green Transportation Options.

For short distances, consider walking or cycling instead of driving. These options not only reduce carbon emissions but also offer health benefits through physical activity.

Creating a Green Community.

Sharing eco-friendly practices with friends, family, and neighbors can create a community that values and practices sustainability. Community gardens, shared composting facilities, and local clean-up drives can foster a sense of togetherness and collective responsibility towards the planet.

A Healthy Home for a Healthy Planet.

Embracing eco-friendly practices in our homes is a step towards personal health and planetary well-being. It's about making conscious choices that respect and preserve nature. In doing so, we not only create healthier living spaces but also contribute to a more sustainable world.

Gut Health: Foods and Tips for a Healthy Microbiome.

The gut plays a pivotal role in overall health. A healthy gut microbiome is not just about digestion; it's a cornerstone of well-being, influencing everything from mood to immunity. Here's a journey into understanding the microbiome and how to nourish it with wisdom both ancient and new.

Understanding the Microbiome.

The gut microbiome is a complex ecosystem of bacteria, fungi, and viruses living in our digestive system. These microorganisms are not just passengers; they're instrumental in digesting food, producing vitamins, and even regulating the immune system. A balanced microbiome is key to good health.

Fermented Foods: A Traditional Treasure.

Fermented foods are a gift from our ancestors. Foods like yogurt, kefir, sauerkraut, and kimchi are rich in probiotics, the good bacteria that replenish our gut flora. Incorporating these into daily meals can be a delightful adventure in both taste and health.

Fiber-Rich Foods: The Gut's Best Friend.

Fiber acts as a prebiotic, providing the necessary nutrients for probiotics to thrive. Vegetables, fruits, legumes, and whole grains are excellent sources. A colorful plate not only pleases the eye but also feeds the gut.

Hydration: The Unsung Hero.

Water is essential for gut health. It aids in digestion and helps maintain the balance of good bacteria. Herbal teas can be a soothing addition, offering hydration with a hint of nature's best.

Mindful Eating: The Art of Awareness.

How we eat is as important as what we eat. Mindful eating, a concept deeply rooted in traditional practices, involves eating slowly and savoring every bite. This not only enhances digestion but also brings a sense of calm and contentment.

Stress Reduction: Calm the Mind, Heal the Gut.

Stress can disrupt gut health. Practices like meditation, gentle yoga, and spending time in nature can reduce stress levels. Barbara O'Neil often spoke about the interconnection of mind and body health, emphasizing relaxation for overall well-being.

Avoiding Gut Aggressors.

Processed foods, high in sugar and unhealthy fats, can disrupt the microbiome. Limiting these and opting for whole, unprocessed foods can prevent the imbalance of gut bacteria.

Gut-Friendly Cooking: A Joyful Journey.

Cooking for gut health doesn't have to be a chore. Experimenting with different herbs, spices, and fresh ingredients can turn meal preparation into a joyful journey of discovery.

Regular Exercise: Keep Moving for a Healthy Gut.

Physical activity is beneficial for the gut. It enhances gut motility and diversity of the microbiome. Even a daily brisk walk can make a difference.

Sleep: The Regenerative Power.

Adequate sleep is crucial for gut health. It's during sleep that the body repairs itself, which includes balancing the microbiome. Developing a regular sleep routine can have profound effects on gut health.

Community and Connection

Sharing meals and connecting with others can also contribute to gut health. The act of eating in a pleasant, social environment can positively affect digestion and absorption of nutrients.

A Holistic Approach to Gut Health.

Caring for the gut is a holistic endeavor. It's about more than just food; it's about lifestyle choices that encompass mind, body, and spirit. Taking on these practices can lead to a vibrant microbiome and, consequently, a healthier, happier life.

STRESS-FREE LIVING: PRACTICAL EVERYDAY STRATEGIES.

Stress has become as common as the air we breathe. Yet, in the whispers of nature and the wisdom of traditional practices, we find timeless strategies to ease our daily stresses. Barbara O'Neil often emphasized the importance of creating a stress-free environment through simple, everyday actions. Here's a guide to infusing tranquility into your daily life, blending age-old wisdom with practical modern strategies.

THE POWER OF MORNING RITUALS.

Start your day with a peaceful ritual. Whether it's a few moments of deep breathing, a gentle yoga session, or a quiet cup of herbal tea, these activities set a calm tone for the day. Just as the sun rises gently, allow your day to begin softly, gradually building momentum.

NURTURING WITH NATURE.

Nature is a formidable healer. Spending time outdoors, whether it's a walk in the park, gardening, or simply sitting under a tree, can significantly reduce stress levels. The Japanese practice of Shinrin-yoku or 'forest bathing' is a testament to the calming power of being in nature.

MINDFUL EATING FOR MINDFUL LIVING.

Mealtimes are not just for nourishment but also for relaxation. Eating slowly, savoring each bite, and being thankful for the food can transform a simple meal into a peaceful experience. Avoid eating on the go or while distracted; instead, make each meal a mindful act.

THE ART OF 'DOING NOTHING'.

In a world that glorifies busyness, doing nothing can be revolutionary. Set aside time each day to simply be. Sit quietly, gaze out of the window, or listen to calming music. This practice of 'doing nothing' can be surprisingly rejuvenating.

DIGITAL DETOX.

Technology, while beneficial, can also be a source of stress. Allocate certain times of the day to disconnect from digital devices. This digital detox can help reduce anxiety and improve focus and sleep quality.

BREATHWORK: THE SIMPLEST STRESS RELIEVER.

Deep breathing exercises are a quick and effective way to alleviate stress. Techniques like the 4-7-8 method or diaphragmatic breathing can be done anywhere and have an immediate calming effect.

PRIORITIZE SLEEP.

A good night's sleep is crucial for stress management. Develop a calming bedtime routine, perhaps including a warm bath, reading, or gentle stretches. Ensure your bedroom is a sanctuary of peace, conducive to restful sleep.

CULTIVATING GRATITUDE.

Gratitude shifts focus from what is lacking to what is abundant. Keeping a gratitude journal or simply reflecting on a few things you're grateful for each day can uplift your mood and reduce stress.

Physical Activity as a Stress Buster.

Exercise releases endorphins, known as the body's natural stress relievers. Incorporate some form of physical activity into your daily routine, be it a brisk walk, a dance session, or a bike ride.

Connect with Others.

Social connections can act as a buffer against stress. Spend time with loved ones, engage in community activities, or simply share a laugh with a friend. Remember, human connection is a key ingredient in the recipe for a stress-free life.

Learn to Say No.

Setting boundaries is vital for managing stress. It's okay to say no to additional responsibilities or social engagements if they cause anxiety or overwhelm.

Creating a Cozy Environment.

Your surroundings can significantly impact your mood. Create a cozy, clutter-free environment at home with elements like soft lighting, comfortable furniture, and plants. A harmonious space promotes a harmonious mind.

Embracing a Stress-Free Life.

Living stress-free is not about eliminating challenges but about managing them with grace and wisdom. With these simple yet effective strategies in everyday life, you can navigate through life's complexities with ease and tranquility. A peaceful life begins with peaceful moments. Choose calm, choose serenity, choose a stress-free life.

THE ART OF FERMENTATION: PROBIOTICS FOR GUT HEALTH.

In the quest for gut health, the age-old practice of fermentation emerges as a delightful blend of culinary art and wellness science. This process, rooted in tradition yet embraced by modern health enthusiasts, transforms everyday foods into probiotic powerhouses. It's a journey into the heart of natural health, where the simplicity of fermentation meets the complexity of the gut microbiome.

UNVEILING THE MAGIC OF MICROBES.

Fermentation is an excellent twist of microorganisms, primarily bacteria and yeast, which convert sugars and starches in foods into alcohol or acids. This natural alchemy not only preserves the food but also creates a host of beneficial probiotics, enzymes, and vitamins.

A NOD TO ANCESTRAL WISDOM.

Fermentation is a testament to the wisdom of our ancestors. Traditional cultures around the world have long harnessed the power of fermentation, not just to preserve food but also for its health-enhancing properties. From sauerkraut in Germany to kimchi in Korea, these fermented delights are more than just culinary heritage; they are time-honored remedies for a healthy gut.

THE PROBIOTIC POWER: A GUT HEALTH ALLY.

The probiotics generated through fermentation are friendly bacteria that play a crucial role in gut health. They aid digestion, boost the immune system, and may even improve mental health. Using fermented foods in daily meals is an easy and natural way to nurture the gut microbiome, fostering a balance that is essential for overall well-being.

FERMENTATION AT HOME: A FUN AND HEALTHY HOBBY.

Embracing fermentation is not just about consuming probiotics; it's about engaging in a gratifying process that connects us to our food in a meaningful way. Here's how to start:

- Choose Your Base: Vegetables like cabbage, carrots, and cucumbers are great for beginners. Dairy enthusiasts can try fermenting milk to make yogurt or kefir.

- Add Salt or a Starter Culture: Salt inhibits harmful bacteria, allowing beneficial bacteria to flourish. For dairy ferments, specific starter cultures are required.

- Create the Right Environment: Most ferments do well in a cool, dark place. An airtight container is essential to create an anaerobic environment.

- Patience is Key: Fermentation is a slow process. The transformation from raw ingredients to fermented foods can take days to weeks.

- Experiment and Enjoy: The beauty of fermentation lies in its versatility. Experiment with different ingredients and flavors to create unique blends.

FERMENTED FOODS: A GATEWAY TO CREATIVE COOKING.

Incorporating fermented foods into daily meals can be a delightful culinary adventure. Here are a few ideas:

Sauerkraut as a Side Dish: A classic fermented cabbage, perfect alongside meats or in sandwiches.

Kimchi in Stir-fries: This spicy Korean staple can add a zesty twist to stir-fries or rice dishes.

Kefir in Smoothies: A probiotic-rich alternative to yogurt, kefir makes a great base for smoothies.

Miso in Soups: A traditional Japanese seasoning, miso adds depth and flavor to soups and broths.

FERMENTATION AS A LIFESTYLE CHOICE.

The art of fermentation is more than just a method of food preservation; it's a lifestyle choice that promotes health, creativity, and a deeper connection with the natural world. It's a delightful journey into the heart of culinary tradition, where each jar of fermented food is not just a source of probiotics but a symbol of the enduring wisdom of nature and nutrition. In embracing fermentation, one doesn't just nourish the gut; one also revives an age-old tradition, crafting delicious, healthful foods that are as enjoyable to make as they are to eat.

Natural Strategies for Hormonal Balance.

Hormones play a leading role in our body system. They are the chemical messengers orchestrating critical aspects of our well-being, from mood to metabolism. Yet, hormonal imbalances are becoming increasingly common, leading to a plethora of health issues. Fortunately, nature offers a bounty of solutions to restore this delicate balance.

Understanding the Hormonal Symphony.

Hormones are produced by various glands in the body and influence almost every cell, organ, and function. They regulate everything from growth and development to how we respond to stress and how our body breaks down food. When this complex system is out of tune, it can have profound effects on our overall health.

Diet: The First Step to Harmony.

What we eat plays a pivotal role in hormonal health. Certain foods can help balance hormones, while others can exacerbate imbalances. Nutrient-rich, whole foods are the cornerstones of a hormone-friendly diet. Foods high in Omega-3 fatty acids, like flaxseeds and fish, support hormone production. Leafy greens and cruciferous vegetables, rich in antioxidants and fiber, aid in detoxification and estrogen balance.

The Power of Herbs and Supplements.

Nature's pharmacy offers an array of herbs known for their hormone-balancing properties. Adaptogens, like Ashwagandha and Rhodiola, help the body adapt to stress, a significant disruptor of hormonal balance. Chaste tree berry (Vitex) is renowned for its ability to regulate menstrual cycles and improve fertility. For men, saw palmetto supports prostate health and testosterone levels.

Stress Management: A Key to Hormonal Equilibrium.

Stress is a major contributor to hormonal imbalance, particularly in the secretion of cortisol, the stress hormone. Engaging in stress-reduction practices like yoga, meditation, and deep breathing exercises can significantly improve hormonal health.

Sleep: The Unsung Hero of Hormonal Health.

Inadequate sleep disrupts the balance of key hormones like cortisol, insulin, and growth hormone. Establishing a regular sleep schedule and creating a restful environment free from electronic devices can foster hormone regulation.

Exercise: Movement as Medicine.

Regular physical activity is crucial for hormonal health. It reduces insulin levels and increases insulin sensitivity. Exercise also boosts mood-enhancing hormones like endorphins. It doesn't have to be intense; even daily walks and gentle yoga can have significant benefits.

Environmental Toxins and Hormones.

Exposure to certain chemicals in our environment can disrupt hormonal function. These endocrine disruptors, found in plastics, personal care products, and pesticides, mimic hormones and confuse our body's natural hormonal signaling. Opting for organic foods and natural, eco-friendly products can reduce this risk.

Barbara O'Neil's Teachings and Hormonal Health.

Barbara O'Neil, a noted naturopath, emphasizes the importance of a holistic approach to health. Her teachings align with the principles of hormonal balance, advocating for a diet rich in whole foods, the healing power of herbs, and the necessity of managing stress and getting quality sleep.

A Journey to Hormonal Harmony.

Hormonal balance is not a destination but a continuous journey of mindful choices. It's about tuning into our body's natural rhythms and providing it with the support it needs through diet, lifestyle, and a connection with nature. This journey, while uniquely personal, is universally grounded in the wisdom of nature and our ancestors, offering a timeless solution to a modern challenge.

Conclusion.

As we reach the end of this enlightening journey in Volume 1 of our exploration into natural wellness and home remedies, it's time to reflect on the wealth of knowledge we've gathered. We've ventured through a remarkable array of topics, each opening a door to a deeper understanding of how nature and simple, everyday items can significantly contribute to our health and well-being.

We began with the surprising benefits of "Onion Socks: An Unexpected Cold Remedy," unraveling the age-old wisdom hidden in our kitchens. This led us to discover the "Quick At-Home Teeth Whitening Secret," showcasing how simple ingredients can bring out our brightest smiles.

Our journey took us through nutrition and natural beauty, from "Tasty Salads That Naturally Aid Weight Loss" to "Natural Hair Care: Herbal Secrets for Healthy Locks." We learned how beetroot and sweet potatoes, humble yet powerful, can transform our health in "Beetroot's Hidden Benefits for Blood Pressure and Energy" and "The Little-Known Health Benefits of Sweet Potatoes."

"Revitalizing Meals: Quick and Healthy Recipes" and "Detoxifying Natural Weight Loss Drinks" opened our eyes to the simplicity and joy of cooking with nature's bounty. We went further into the uses of household items in "Baking Soda Wonders: From Cleaning to Health" and "Polyethylene Bags: Surprising Household Uses," finding new appreciation for these everyday objects.

The book guided us through the therapeutic world of "Soothing Herbal Teas for Relaxation and Health" and the practical strategies in "Stress-Free Living: Practical Everyday Strategies." Each page turned was a step towards understanding how to harmoniously intertwine our lives with the rhythm of nature.

We discovered the power of mindfulness in "Meditation for Everyday Calm" and "Mindful Eating: Transforming Your Relationship with Food," learning how awareness can profoundly impact our health. "Yoga for Every Body: Flexibility and Strength" and "The Trampoline Workout: Fun Fitness Revolution" brought fun and innovation into our fitness routines.

Exploring "Eco-Friendly Home Practices for Health" and "Travel Wellness: Staying Healthy on the Go," we expanded our horizons beyond the confines of our homes, learning to maintain our wellness wherever life takes us.

Still, this is merely the beginning. Our exploration in Volume 1 has laid a strong foundation of knowledge and practices, but there is still so much more to discover. The world of natural health and wellness is vast and ever-evolving, and as we close this volume, we do so with anticipation and excitement for the continuing journey.

Stay tuned for Volume 2, where we will launch into even more intriguing and beneficial topics. We'll search the ancient practices of Ayurveda, uncover the secrets of essential oils, and learn about the wonders of hydrotherapy. Expect to discuss subjects like "The Healing Power of Music and Sound Therapy," "Urban Gardening: Growing Your Own Health," and "The Magic of Mushrooms: A Superfood Spotlight." We'll also look at "Mind-Body Connection: Techniques for Inner Harmony" and "Seasonal Eating: Aligning Diet with Nature's Rhythms."

The journey to holistic health and natural wellness is ongoing, and there's always more to learn, practice, and explore. Thank you for joining this journey in Volume 1, and may you carry its lessons and insights with you as you continue to nurture your health and well-being in harmony with nature. Stay curious, stay inspired, and be ready to embark on the next phase of this adventure with Volume 2.

As we close the first volume of our journey into the world of natural wellness and home remedies, the path ahead beckons with even more fascinating discoveries. In Volume 2, we will sink deeper into the art of living in harmony with nature, uncovering age-old secrets and modern insights that promise to enhance your health and well-being.

Prepare to be captivated by the revival of "Traditional Remedies for Modern Ailments," where ancient wisdom meets contemporary health challenges. Imagine harnessing the "Healing Power of Sunshine and Fresh Air," tapping into nature's most fundamental elements for profound wellness benefits.

We will look at the crucial "Role of Micro-Organisms in Health and Disease," a journey that will change your perspective on these tiny, yet mighty, life forms. For those seeking relief, "Soothing Natural Solutions for Skin Conditions" will offer gentle yet effective ways to care for your skin using the bounty of nature.

Herbal enthusiasts will be delighted with "Herbal Teas: Nature's Answer to Stress and Anxiety," where each sip brings a sense of calm and clarity. Women will find a treasure trove of knowledge in "Natural Approaches to Women's Health Issues," covering everything from hormonal balance to nurturing self-care practices.

Parents will find invaluable insights in "Children's Health: Natural Tips for Growing Bodies," ensuring the little ones grow up with the best that nature can offer. And for everyone looking to cleanse and rejuvenate, "Detoxifying Your Body: Safe and Effective Methods" will guide you through gentle, natural detoxification practices.

Volume 2 also examines the "Miracle of Plant-Based Eating for Health," unraveling the power of a diet rich in fruits, vegetables, and whole grains. Fitness enthusiasts will discover "Exercise Essentials: Natural Ways to Enhance Fitness," blending ancient practices with modern exercise science.

The journey continues with topics like "Natural Remedies for Allergy Relief," "Heart Health: Natural Ways to Nourish Your Heart," and "The Healing Power of Aromatherapy." Each chapter opens up new possibilities for healing and wellness, grounded in the wisdom of nature and the body's innate healing abilities.

"Natural First Aid: Preparing for Minor Injuries" will equip you with the knowledge to handle everyday bumps and bruises naturally. We'll also explore "The Role of Fasting in Health and Healing," examining how strategic fasting can rejuvenate your body and mind.

You will also be intrigued by "Holistic Approaches to Diabetes Management" and discover "The Healing Properties of Common Spices" that you can find in your kitchen. For those struggling with chronic conditions, "Understanding and Managing Chronic Diseases Naturally" will offer hope and practical strategies.

As we go through this continuation of our wellness journey, Volume 2 promises to be an essential companion for anyone passionate about embracing a natural, holistic approach to health. It's not just a collection of tips and remedies; it's a guide to living a life that's in tune with nature's rhythms and wisdom. So stay curious, keep exploring, and let's together unlock the doors to a healthier, happier life with the upcoming

The End.
Margaret Willowbrook.

Further Resources for Exploration

Barbara O'Neill Resources:

- **YouTube Lectures and Seminars:** Search for Barbara O'Neill on YouTube to find numerous lectures and seminars where she discusses topics related to health, nutrition, and natural remedies.

- **Health and Wellness Websites:** Look for articles featuring Barbara O'Neill on well-known health and wellness platforms. While specific URLs can't be provided, websites like Healthline or Natural News often feature articles by or about health experts.

- **Books:** Barbara O'Neill has authored several books on health and wellness. A search on online bookstores like Amazon or Barnes & Noble may provide you with titles available for purchase or download.

- **Podcasts:** There are health and wellness podcasts that may feature interviews with Barbara O'Neill. Platforms like Spotify and Apple Podcasts are good places to start searching.

General Health and Wellness Resources:

- **PubMed:** For scientific articles and studies related to health, nutrition, and fitness topics, PubMed is a free search engine accessing the MEDLINE database of citations and abstracts.

- **Google Scholar:** Another excellent resource for academic papers, thesis, books, and conference papers on a wide range of subjects including health and wellness.

- **WebMD (webmd.com):** Offers a wealth of health information, tools for managing your health, and support to those who seek information.

- **Mayo Clinic (mayoclinic.org):** A nonprofit organization committed to clinical practice, education, and research, providing expert, whole-person care to everyone who needs healing.

- **Healthline (healthline.com):** Provides health and wellness information that's authoritative and approachable. By understanding the facts, you can make the best decisions for your health.

- **Medical News Today (medicalnewstoday.com):** Offers detailed articles on a wide range of health topics, news, and research findings.

- **MindBodyGreen (mindbodygreen.com):** Focuses on connecting soul and science, with articles on wellness, nutrition, and personal growth.

- **The Nutrition Source (The Nutrition Source):** Provided by the Harvard T.H. Chan School of Public Health, offering evidence-based guidance on nutrition.

- **Examine.com (examine.com):** Independent and unbiased source on nutrition and supplements, providing research-based information.

- **ACE Fitness (acefitness.org):** The American Council on Exercise offers fitness certifications and valuable information on exercise, nutrition, and the latest fitness trends.

- **Precision Nutrition (precisionnutrition.com):** Offers in-depth articles on nutrition and coaching for fitness professionals and enthusiasts.

- **Yoga Journal (yogajournal.com):** Provides all things yoga, including poses, meditation guides, and the benefits of yoga practice for physical and mental health.

A MESSAGE FROM THE PUBLISHER:

Are you enjoying the book? We would love to hear your thoughts!

Many readers do not know how hard reviews are to come by and how much they help a publisher. We would be incredibly grateful if you could take just a few seconds to write a brief review on Amazon, even if it's just a few sentences!

Please go here to leave a quick review:

https://amazon.com/review/create-review?&asin=B0CV83455J

We would greatly appreciate it if you could take the time to post your review of the book and share your thoughts with the community. If you have enjoyed the book, please let us know what you loved the most about it and if you would recommend it to others. Your feedback is valuable to us, and it helps us to improve our services and continue to offer high-quality literature to our readers.

Made in the USA
Columbia, SC
14 July 2024